MEAL PREP

The Complete Meal Prep Guide for Batch Cooking, Weight Loss and Clean Eating – Includes 60+ Low Carb Keto Recipes

© Copyright 2017 by Tyler Smith- All rights reserved.

The following book is reproduced below with the goal of providing information that is as accurate and as reliable as possible. Regardless, purchasing this book can be seen as consent to the fact that both the publisher and the author of this book are in no way experts on the topics discussed within, and that any recommendations or suggestions made herein are for entertainment purposes only. Professionals should be consulted as needed before undertaking any of the action endorsed herein.

This declaration is deemed fair and valid by both the American Bar Association and the Committee of Publishers Association and is legally binding throughout the United States.

Furthermore, the transmission, duplication or reproduction of any of the following work, including precise information, will be considered an illegal act, irrespective whether it is done electronically or in print. The legality extends to creating a secondary or tertiary copy of the work or a recorded copy and is only allowed with express written consent of the Publisher. All additional rights are reserved.

The information in the following pages is broadly considered to be a truthful and accurate account of facts, and as such any inattention, use or misuse of the information in question by the reader will render any resulting actions solely under their purview. There are no scenarios in which the publisher or the original author of this work can be in any fashion deemed liable for any hardship or damages that may befall them after undertaking information described herein.

Additionally, the information found on the following pages is intended for informational purposes only and should thus be considered, universal. As befitting its nature, the information presented is without assurance regarding its continued validity or interim quality. Trademarks that mentioned are done without written consent and can in no way be considered an endorsement from the trademark holder.

Table of Contents

Introduction 1

Chapter 1: Meal Prepping Hacks and Ideas 2

Chapter 2: Novice Meal Prepping Mistakes to Avoid 11

Chapter 3: Helpful Equipment 14

Chapter 4 Calories, Nutrition, Macronutrients, and Micronutrient 18

Chapter 5: Chicken and Beef Keto-Rich Recipes 23

Chapter 7: Seafood Recipes That Are Low in Carbs 41

Chapter 7: Healthy Soups for Slurping 57

Chapter 8: Salads Recipes So Good You'll Forget You're Eating One 75

Chapter 9: Vegan Dishes for the Compassionate Heart 91

Conclusion 104

INTRODUCTION

Congratulations on getting your personal copy of *Meal Prep: The Complete Meal Prep Guide for Batch Cooking, Weight Loss and Clean Eating – Includes 60+ Low Carb Keto Recipes*.

The following chapters will provide you with information on how you can cook in larger quantities and then divide these quantities into portioned weekly meals. In addition to learning about how you can save yourself time in the kitchen with batch cooking, this book will also provide you with recipes that are low in carbs and healthy in nature. After reading this book, it's more than likely that you will feel motivated to at least start thinking about how you can best integrate batch cooking healthy meals into your weekly lifestyle. It's safe to say that most people do not entirely enjoy coming home from work with the knowledge that they will have to cook a meal for themselves. With batch cooking, all you have to do with your meal is take it out of the refrigerator and heat it up. That's why batch cooking matters.

Again, thank you for getting your own personal copy of *Meal Prep: The Complete Meal Prep Guide for Batch Cooking, Weight Loss and Clean Eating – Includes 60+ Low Carb Keto Recipes*. Enjoy the rest of what this book has to offer you.

Chapter 1
Meal Prepping Hacks and Ideas

In case you have not yet read my other book on meal prepping, meal prepping can be briefly defined as prepping your meals in advanced so that you can better adhere to a certain meal plan or meal schedule. People choose to prep their meals for a variety of reasons. Since you're reading this book, it's likely that you plan on prepping recipes that are low in carbs. While my other book has already gone over the many benefits that meal prepping can provide for an individual's life, this chapter is going to look at some of the more detailed nuances of meal prepping. After reading this chapter, you're going to have a subtler understanding of some of the less-discussed, yet still incredibly important, meal prepping tactics that you should be keeping in mind as you move towards a new lifestyle change for yourself.

Start with Your Worst Habit

Initially, it may seem daunting to think about prepping all of the meals that you're going to consume for the entire week in a single period of time. It is normal to feel this way. If you want to start your journey with meal prepping on a smaller scale, you should take some time to think about your current worst meal habit. For example, if you know deep down that you don't cook breakfast for yourself during the week because there's a Starbuck's conveniently located right next to your office, start there. If you have a bad habit of eating out with coworkers during your lunch hour, maybe this is where you need to start. Whatever your habit is, recognize it and change it. Not only will this allow you to curb your daily spending, it will also slowly entice you to become more disciplined when it comes to eating predetermined and healthy meals.

Use Any Spare Time that You Have

We're all busy people. Another reason why individuals who are new to meal prepping often feel a tad overwhelmed when they're first getting started is because they feel as if they don't have the time to be spending hours in the kitchen prepping meals. This is a fair assessment; however, your lack of time does not mean that you should give up entirely. If we think about eating as more of a habit than anything else, then it becomes clear that the way in which you prepare your meals is just as important as the types of foods that you're consuming. Even if you can't find the time to prep all of your meals for the week in a single day, you should still do what you can. For example, prep your snacks that you're going to take with you to work, or prep only your lunches for the week. By slowing down and planning any of your meals, it's more likely that you will gradually work towards eventually finding the time to prep all of your meals for the week.

Find Your Staple Recipes

After you've prepped your meals for a couple of weeks, you should seek to identify the meals that are the most fulfilling when it comes to both efficient meal prepping and quenching your appetite. Once you've identified these few recipes, you should plan to integrate them into your weekly meal prepping more often. Doing this will achieve two things. One, it will allow you to feel more comfortable in the kitchen. If you've already prepped something a few times before, it's going to feel easier than attempting a recipe that you've never tried before. This will help to build your meal prepping confidence. Two, staple recipes will allow you to become more comfortable when it comes time to add some variety to your meal prepping process.

Make Sure Your Containers Match

If you've ever purchased Tupperware in the past, then you already know that sometimes it can be a tricky and time-consuming task to locate the correct lid for the Tupperware that you're looking to use during a given period of time. If your meal prepping containers are unorganized, how do you expect to be efficient in the kitchen? It may seem silly, but many people who have been meal prepping for quite some time attest to the fact that being organized with your containers is an important part of the entire meal prepping process. Two pieces of advice that you should seek to follow in regards to your containers include the following:

1. **Buy the same types of meal prep containers.** Trying out different containers might seem fun, but it's not going to be fun when you're unable to match your lids with your containers when you're in a hurry.

2. **Match Your Lids and Containers Up Right Away:** As soon as you remove your containers from the dishwasher, take the time to match them together as soon as possible. If they're not dry when they're removed from the dishwasher, you don't want to seal the lid to the container, as this could lead to moisture and mold accumulation. Instead, stack all similar lids and all similar containers together. This will allow you to easily figure out what goes with what.

Vegetables

One of the most tedious ingredients to prepare when you are cooking is the vegetables. Dishes may require a different way of cutting the vegetables. Some of them have to be julienned, diced, minced, wedged, cubed, shredded, or spiraled.

The way the vegetables are cut or prepared will affect their shelf time. The larger the cut, the longer they could stay fresh. It also depends on the vegetable. Cruciferous or hard vegetables can stay fresh longer, while soft and acidic vegetables may not last more than three days. Below is the freshness time table of some vegetables:

Vegetable	Cut	Freshness Time in the Fridge
Onions	Sliced/minced	3 days. It should be stored in a dry container and sealed tightly.
	Peeled, whole	7 days. It should be wrapped tightly in a cling wrap.
Squash (any variety)	Cubed, uncooked	5 days. Make sure to keep it in a dry Ziploc plastic and remove as much air as possible. Use a vacuum sealer if you have one.
	Cubed, cooked	5 days, if roasted separately from other vegetables. 3 days if roasted with other vegetables or poached.
Potatoes/Sweet Potatoes	Whole, peeled	3 days. Make sure that it is dry and wrapped tightly in cling wrap.

	Julienned, cubed	3 days. Make sure that the container is dry and no moisture can enter.
	whole, roasted	5 days. Keep it wrapped in aluminum foil and sealed in a container or Ziploc. Make sure to cool it down first before storing.
Zucchini	Julienned, cubed, shredded	5 days. Pack it in a sealed bag.
	Whole, raw or roasted	5 days. Pack it tightly in a cling wrap. If it is roasted, make sure to cool it first.
Spinach and other leafy vegetables	Shredded, torn	5 days. You should pack it in a perforated plastic.
	Whole, with stem	7 days. Wash the vegetable. Wrap it in a paper towel and place in perforated plastic.
Celery	Sliced and cubed	7 days, when vacuumed sealed. 3 to 5 days, when it is packed dry in a Ziploc.
	Whole	2 weeks. Remove as much moisture as possible.
Cauliflower and Broccoli	Whole	1 week. Wrap it tightly in cling wrap.

	Sliced	3 to 5 days. Make sure that the container or the Ziploc bag is dry.
	Sliced and roasted or pre-cooked	3 days. Make sure to cool it before packing. You should not let the vegetable get into contact with moisture. Also, do not roast it along with vegetables that have more moisture, like carrots, squash, and zucchini.
Carrots	Julienned, shredded, cubed	1 week. Pack it in a sealed container.
	Whole	1 week. Dry the carrot first before wrapping it in cling wrap.
Garlic	Minced, chopped, pureed	2 days. Store it in a glass container and keep it in a dark portion of the fridge.
	Whole cloves	5 days. Store in a dry, sealed plastic.
Pepper	Julienned, sliced	3 days. Pack it in a dry container or plastic.
	Whole	A week. Make sure to place it somewhere with minimal moisture.
	Whole, roasted	3 days. Keep it wrapped in aluminum foil and sealed in a container.

Asparagus	Whole	5 to 7 days. Keep in a perforated bag
	Whole, roasted	3 to 5 days. Do not remove from the aluminum foil and keep it in a sealed plastic.
Cabbage	Whole	A week, if wrapped tightly in cling wrap.
	Torn and separated	5 days. Put it in a perforated bag.
	Shredded or julienned	3 days. Keep it in a dry container. Do not introduce moisture as much as possible.
Fresh leafy spices		1 week. Keep them in perforated plastic bags.

Meat and Poultry

Meat and Poultry tend to take a lot of time to cook. An average chicken leg takes 15 minutes to cook (fried or boiled).

Beef steaks may take less time to cook depending on how you want it done. It can take anywhere from 5 minutes to 15 minutes. However, the marinating time can take about 20 minutes to an hour.

Beef used for stews may take more than three hours to cook.

Cutting down the cooking time of these meats is actually easy. You can pre-cook them and store them in the fridge for 2 to 3 days. You can also pre-marinate the meats for broiling or barbecue, to cut your prep time.

Here are some hacks you might want to try:

1. Marinate and seal your meat. You can place your meat in a Ziploc plastic and pour your favorite marinade. Place it in the fridge and thaw when you need to cook it.

2. If you have a vacuum sealer, you can marinade your meat for at least an hour. Remove the excess marinade and vacuum seal it. The juice and the marinade would seep into the meat while being sealed.

3. Pre-roast the chicken. Roasted chicken has a lot of use. You can use it as a main dish. You just have to pop it back in the microwave for 3 to 5 minutes. You can also use it for making sandwiches, soups, and salads.

4. Pre-boil meat that should be used for stew. If you want to include braised beef or chicken in your meal plan, you can boil the meat with salt and pepper until it is soft and tender. Cool it down and pack it in a tightly-sealed container or cling wrap. Freeze the stock.

Fish

Stocking Fish

Fish are faster to cook. You may not have to pre-cook them or pre-marinade them. When stocking fish, consider some of these tips:

1. Cover the cleaned fish with thick cling wrap and freeze it.

2. When you are buying fish steaks, ask the personnel to vacuum seal it for you. If you have your own vacuum sealer,

seal it. Sealing is among the best means of keeping the flavor intact.

Preparing Fish

If you do not have that much time to prepare and cook your fish, you can try to prepare it beforehand by making pappilote. It's the practice of wrapping fish in aluminum foil or parchment.

You can assemble it by wrapping fish with added salt and pepper. When you are about to cook it, just throw in some vegetables and sprinkle olive oil on the fish. Bake it for at least 10 minutes.

There are some other pappilote recipes that you can try in the chapter about seafood.

Chapter 2
Novice Meal Prepping Mistakes to Avoid

Now that you're aware of some of the more nuanced tactics that you can use when you're preparing to meal prep, we are now going to turn our attention to mistakes that you can avoid while prepping meals in the kitchen. This chapter is not meant to intimidate you; rather, it's meant to provide you with insight that should prevent you from making these same common mistakes yourself. In recognizing and discussing these mistakes, the hope is that you will notice when you're about to make one of them and then avoid the hassle of the mistake altogether.

Meal Prepping Mistake 1: Figuring Out Your Recipes on the Fly

One of the most common mistakes that new meal preppers can make is that they don't take the time that's needed to figure out the recipes that they're going to be prepping for the rest of the week. By waiting until the last minute to think about what's going to be prepped for the following week, you're setting yourself up for unnecessary hassle in multiple ways. For one, waiting until the last-minute means that your grocery list is likely to be missing key ingredients, causing you to waste time by having to go to the grocery store multiple times. Another potential byproduct of this mistake involves not fully understanding the meal prep steps that are involved. Remember, you're going to be cooking multiple meals simultaneously. If you don't plan how you're going to utilize the space in your kitchen properly, redundancy is much more likely.

A great way to avoid the potential problems that were discussed above is to create a system that you're going to use in order to find and plan your recipe process. Some people do this by perusing recipe books on a certain day of the week before work in the mornings. Others do this by doing research on the internet and finding recipes that are foolproof and taste good too. Whatever your method may be, it's important to create one and get in the habit of fully understanding what your meal prep process is going to be prior to the day that you're going to meal prep.

Meal Prepping Mistake 2: You Don't Think About Your Food's Aesthetic

Even though your food may look delicious the day that you prep it, once you prep it and put in your refrigerator, it could end up looking less aesthetically pleasing after a couple of days. When your food doesn't look "pretty", it can become more difficult to consume it. A great tip that can help you to keep your food looking good even after its first been prepped is to utilize a cast iron skillet. This type of grill pan will allow you to scorch the sides of your proteins and vegetables with its signature black lines, and will keep your food looking appealing for days. This may seem like an inconsequential detail in regards in meal prepping, but when you're eating similar foods day in and day out, aesthetics tend to matter a bit more than they did when you were eating out more often.

Meal Prepping Mistake 3: Working Until It's Finished

It's safe to say that no one wants to spend their entire day cooking food; however, when you first start to meal prep you may realize that what you originally anticipate to only take a couple of hours can end up taking most of your day. Another common mistake that many novice meal preppers fall into is working until all of the work is done. Yes, setting goals for yourself is always a good thing, but if you misinterpret a recipe or miscalculate the amount of time it's going to take you to finish your prepping, you don't want to be paying for it for the rest of the day.

Instead of thinking of meal prepping as something that needs to be done to completion, it might be a more realistic goal to set a timer for yourself while you're prepping. For example, if you dedicate three hours to meal prepping on a certain day, you can set a timer and work for those three full hours. This will allow you to appreciate the work that you did complete. It will also prevent you from feeling overwhelmed when something doesn't go quite as you initially planned.

Meal Prepping Mistake 4: Not Utilizing All of Your Tools to the Fullest Extent Possible

Lastly, it's important to take shortcuts while you're meal prepping when you can. For example, if you know that you're going to be cooking rice more often, why not invest in a rice cooker? If a recipe calls for cooking something for a longer period of time, it might make sense to invest in a slow cooker. Other types of appliances that will certainly come in handy when it comes to meal prep include food processors, blenders, and maybe even a scale so that you can make portion calculations more accurately. If you're serious about improving your eating habits, then investing some money into these types of appliances should make sense. These tools speed the meal prep process up, yet many novice meal preppers often opt to do without them for some unknown reason.

Chapter 3
Helpful Equipment

Note this equipment is helpful, but not a necessity. Everything can be cooked on a stove, using a skillet, or pots and pans. Knives can be used to cut and plates can function as cutting boards. However, since the point of meal-prep is to save both time and money, these appliances pay for themselves in many ways.

A Crock-pot

This ageless appliance lets you cook and rest at the same time. Although there are only a few crock-pot recipes within these covers, these will not be the only recipes you prepare. If you use a crockpot on cooking day, you can use a larger and less expensive cut of meat. This can be a real savings.

Skillets that are oven proof and non-stick

Most likely if you cook any meals ever you have a skillet or two. In this cookbook, we strive to mess up less dishes. Some of the recipes require browning and then baking. An ovenproof skillet can do both, eliminating one more dish to wash.

At least 3 mixing bowls in large, medium and small sizes

It may be likely that you have these, but not everyone does. As you double or triple recipes when you cook, you will need more than one size and more than one in quantity.

A Blender

Some soups taste better when blended to a creamy puree. It is always easier and tastier to emulsify salad dressings, instead of whipping them by hand in a bowl. You do not have to buy an expensive model as 5 or 6 settings will be enough for the blending instructions we have included.

A Food Processor

When you are preparing multiple meals, using a food processor to chop, slice, and dice saves so much energy and time. The foods are also healthier. Did you know that purchased shredded cheese can include 10 percent wood pulp, commonly called saw dust? When you are purchasing 10 pounds of cheese, you are receiving eight pounds of cheese and two pounds of sawdust. What's more, you are eating it! Save your health by shredding your own blocks of cheese with the food processor. You can freeze it for later use and know the contents of what you are eating.

Good quality sharp knives

Sharp knives make cutting faster and help to keep you from cutting yourself by pressing too hard.

Cutting Boards

Cutting Boards come in several materials and sizes. They protect surfaces and allow the air to circulate underneath while the baked goods cool.

Keep in mind that the construction materials of a cutting board will determine its cleanliness. For example:

Bamboo cutting boards are self-healing. This allows the cuts made by knives to heal on their own. The bamboo cutting boards are very good to knives as they do not dull them quickly. Bamboo is a porous material, which allows bacteria to seep into the cuts. Even disinfecting promptly after use will never eliminate the germs that have accumulated on a wood cutting board.

Plastic boards are non-porous and can be cleaned with stronger chemicals. They still incur cuts and need thorough disinfecting immediately. They will not damage your knives.

Glass cutting boards do not receive cuts, are easy to clean, and can take any kind of chemical disinfectant. They damage knives very quickly and you will be replacing your knives about every three months. Which is less expensive, replacing the cutting boards or the knives?

Glass canning jars with lids, pint sized and quart sized

One of the lesser known secrets is that salad stored in a Ball or Mason jar with a tight sealing lid will stay fresh in the refrigerator for seven full days! This makes the dinner salad, stored in a quart jar, easy to place into serving plates. Salads stored in pint jars are perfect for toting in the thermal lunch bag for a healthy lunch. The salad dressing can be included in the jar and will still be fresh.

Foil containers

These can be expensive, but dollar stores have these priced better than grocery stores. Buy the containers that include lids, baking sizes and the individual sizes.

Plastic containers

Use the food prep containers that are custom designed for Meal-prep. These have no BPAs, are apportioned in the right serving sizes, and are inexpensive. They are dishwasher safe, freezer safe, and can be used in the microwave. Buy enough containers for all your family members to eat three meals a day for one week. You will also need zip-lock freezer bags, pint-sized and snack-sized. Using leftover whipped topping bowls or margarine containers can be less expensive, but they are not constructed to be heated in the microwave or stored for long-term in the freezer.

Chapter 4

Calories, Nutrition, Macronutrients, and Micronutrient

Another important thing to understand in order to make weight loss easier is calories and nutrients. Losing weight is mostly a calorie game. A calorie is a unit of energy and is essential to human health and proper functioning. In fact, you need calories to survive. If you consume just the right amount of calories per day, you'll have enough energy to carry out your daily task. If your calorie consumption is too high, you'll end up packing extra pounds because your body will store the extra energy as fat. This can lead to chronic diseases such as diabetes. If your calorie consumption is low, you'll end up losing weight. However, if your calorie consumption is too low, your vital organs such as your lungs, liver, kidneys, heart, and brain will not function properly. This will also lead to electrolyte imbalances and will decrease your blood sugar and potassium level.

However, weight loss is not just a calorie game. To lose weight and keep your body strong and healthy, you must consume the right kinds of foods. You must eat foods that are rich in both micronutrients and have a correct ratio of macronutrients.

Micronutrients

Micronutrients are vitamins and minerals that play an important role in human growth and development. Although your body only needs a small quantity of each micronutrient, vitamin deficiency can cause serious problems. In fact, in a study published in the Journal of the American College of Nutrition, people lacking in vitamin C, vitamin A, and magnesium are twenty percent more obese than those who consume enough vitamins and minerals.

Micronutrients facilitate growth and help you lose weight by helping in the production of digestive enzymes. They also help rejuvenate your cells and increase your metabolism, helping you look and feel young.

Macronutrients

Macronutrients are nutrients that give your body energy. You need to consume large amounts of these nutrients every day to function well. There are three types of macronutrients – protein, fat, and carbohydrates. To translate the macronutrients into calories:

- 1 gram of carbohydrates = 4 calories
- 1 gram of fat = 9 calories
- 1 gram of protein = 4 calories

Protein

Protein is the building block of all cells in your body. It is made of compounds called amino acids. Your body uses proteins to repair tissues.

On a low-carb keto diet, when you eat high amounts of fat, moderate amount of proteins and only a few carbohydrates, your metabolism changes into a state called ketosis. The protein amount can vary from moderate to high depending on your level of fitness activity. When your body is in a ketosis state, it burns your body fat and converts it to energy. This leads to fat loss.

Eating foods that are rich in protein also suppresses your appetite and helps you lose a lot of water weight.

How much protein should you eat per day? It depends. If you have an active lifestyle, you should consume 0.8-1 grams of protein per pound of weight. For example, if you weigh 150lbs, you should consume 120-150 grams of protein each day.

If you are trying to lose weight, it is also recommended that you consume at least 0.7 grams of protein per pound of weight.

Carbohydrates

Carbohydrates are macronutrients that are made of carbon, hydrogen, and oxygen. There are two types of carbohydrates – simple carbohydrates and complex carbohydrates.

Simple carbohydrates are mainly made of different types of sugars such as glucose, fructose, galactose, lactose, ribose, maltose, galactose, and sucrose. These carbs are easily digested and they provide quick energy that does not last long. They are typically found in desserts, sugar, soda, candies, pastries, and artificial syrups.

Complex carbohydrates are mainly made of starch. They provide longer lasting energy because our bodies take a longer time to break them down into simpler carbs.

Carbs have been getting a lot of bad press from the fitness industry. It's no wonder why more and more people avoid eating carbs. However, carbs are necessary to maintain your body function. You need carbs to carry out physical tasks and help your brain get through a test or task that requires mental prowess. Carbs are useful, but to achieve your weight loss goals, you have to make wise carb choices.

You need carbohydrates to function well. But, some carbohydrates are bad for you and can lead to obesity. This is the reason why it is important to choose the right kinds of carbohydrates. If you want to put your body in a ketosis state and increase your metabolism, you have to limit your calorie intake to 20 to 50 grams per day.

Fats

This macronutrient cushions and protects your organs. It also helps your body absorb vitamins and keeps your skin healthy. Fat stays in your body longer than protein and carbs, and helps you feels satiated. Too much fat can cause obesity, but having enough fat in your body can keep you from binge eating.

There are two common types of fats – saturated and unsaturated fats. Saturated fats are solid at room temperature. These fats can clog your blood vessels and cause various heart diseases.

On the other hand, unsaturated fats are usually found in fish and nuts. They are much healthier for you than saturated fats. Amongst those, are certain types of unsaturated fats called trans fats which are extremely bad for you. Trans fats are the leading cause of heart disease in the United States.

To lose weight and achieve good health, stick to unsaturated fats and try to avoid saturated and trans fats as much as possible.

Your body does need fats to function optimally but you have to choose to consume healthy fats in order for it to do so. For you next meal, skip fried food and eat avocados and nuts instead.

Chapter 5

Chicken and Beef Keto-Rich Recipes

Beef Recipe 1: Ground Beef Zucchini Enchilada Boats

Prep time: 5 minutes; **Cook time:** 35 minutes;
Serving Size: 1.5 zucchini boats; **Serves:** 6;
Calories: 222; **Total Fat:** 10 g; **Protein:** 21 g;
Total Carbs: 11 g; **Net Carbs:** 9 g; **Sugar:** 2 g; **Fiber:** 2 g;

Ingredients:

- 3 zucchinis, cut in half lengthwise with the insides taken out
- 1.5 cups of enchilada sauce
- ¼ cups of cilantro
- ½ cup of Mexican cheese, shredded
- 1 tablespoon of olive oil
- ½ cup of red onion, diced
- 1 pound lean ground beef
- 1 teaspoon of cumin
- 1 teaspoon of paprika
- 2 minced of garlic cloves

Directions:

Heat oven to 350 degrees Fahrenheit. Place a pan on a burner, and cook olive oil and onion for 4 minutes. Next, mix in ground beef. Cook until it's no longer red. Stir in garlic, paprika, and cumin. In a 9 x 9-inch cooking pan, place zucchini shells. Fill with beef, and then cover with enchilada sauce. Top with Mexican cheese blend. Bake for twenty-two minutes. After 22 minutes, remove tin foil from pan and bake for another three minutes. Serve with cilantro on top.

Prep Instructions:

This would best be stored in a plastic meal prep container, with some extra enchilada sauce in the base of the container and cilantro on the side. Keep inside refrigerator for up to 3 days.

Beef Recipe 2: Beefy Taco Pie

Prep time: 15 minutes; **Cook time:** 30 minutes;
Serving Size: 1 waffle; **Serves:** 6;
Calories: 320; **Total Fat:** 21.23 g; **Protein:** 20.17 g
Total Carbs: 2.14 g; **Net Carbs:** 1.95 g; **Sugar:** 0 g; **Fiber:** .19 g;

Ingredients:

- 1 cup of Mexican cheese
- 1 pound of ground beef
- 2 minced of garlic cloves
- 1 cup of whipping cream
- 6 eggs
- ¾ cups of water
- 3 tablespoons of Mexican spice
- ½ teaspoon of salt
- ½ teaspoon of pepper

Directions:

Heat the oven to 400 degrees Fahrenheit. Spray a 9x9-inch pan with non-stick cooking spray. You can also opt to use a pie pan instead of a regular pan. Cook ground beef on your stove top until it's fully cooked-through. Combine Mexican spice to the beef, and then the water. Allow this to simmer for five minutes. Evenly place beef into baking pan. Combine egg, salt, pepper, garlic and whipping cream. Ladle this over the ground beef. Finally, add cheese on top and cook for a half-hour.

Prep Instructions:

If using a pie pan, cut this meal up the same as you would a pizza pie, meaning into 8 equal slices. Place 1-2 slices inside a storage container. Store for up to 5 days without worrying about the meat going bad.

Beef Recipe 3: Salisbury Steak with Mushroom Au Jus

Prep time: 20 minutes; **Cook time:** 20 minutes;
Serving Size: 1 steak & 1/3 cup mushroom au jus; **Serves:** 6;
Calories: 457; **Total Fat:** 24 g; **Protein:** 30 g;
Total Carbs: 5 g; **Net Carbs:** 4.5 g; **Sugar:** .5 g; **Fiber:** .5 g;

Ingredients:

- 2 pounds of lean ground beef
- 3/4 cup of beef broth
- 4 tablespoons of butter
- 1 cup of yellow onions, diced
- ¾ cup flour, almond
- 2 cups mushrooms, any type
- 1 tablespoon of parsley
- ½ teaspoon of garlic powder
- 1.5 teaspoons of salt
- ½ teaspoon of pepper
- ¼ cup of sour cream
- 1.5 tablespoons of Worcestershire

Directions:

Heat oven to 375 degrees Fahrenheit. Mix the beef, almond flour, parsley, ¼ cup of the beef broth, 1 tablespoon Worcestershire, garlic powder, and salt and pepper together. Create patties of steak from the meat mixture that you've made, until well-seasoned and combined. Cook for 20 minutes. While cooking, combine the butter, mushrooms, onions, broth, the rest of the Worcestershire sauce and sour cream. This is going to be your steak's sauce. Cook until everything is combined well and the mushrooms and onions are fully cooked. Drizzle over your steaks once removed from the oven.

Prep Instructions:

Add sauce to every meal prep container. This way, you're guaranteed to get some extra juice on the bottom of each container, and this will help to keep the steak marinated and juicy. 1/3 cup of sauce goes with 1 steak. One steak per meal prep container is plenty. Refrigerate for up 3 days.

Beef Recipe 4: Hamburger & Cauliflower Bake

Prep time: 15 minutes; **Cook time:** 30 minutes;
Serving Size: 1 casserole slice; **Serves:** 6;
Calories: 443; **Total Fat:** 26.8 g; **Protein:** 39 g;
Total Carbs: 16.2 g; **Net Carbs:** 8.7 g; **Sugar:** 1 g; **Fiber:** 7.5 g;

Ingredients:

- 1 cauliflower head
- ¼ cup slivered almonds
- 1 pound of lean ground beef
- ½ teaspoon oregano
- ¼ teaspoon paprika
- ½ teaspoon cumin
- 1 cup milk, coconut
- 2 eggs
- 1 cup chicken broth

Directions:

Heat oven to 350 degrees Fahrenheit. Break the head of the cauliflower up into bits, and steam for about eight minutes. While the cauliflower is cooking, cook the beef in a pan and mix your spices into the pan, too. Once cooked through, set aside. In another bowl, mix eggs, milk, and brother together. Starting with the ground beef, layer a 13x9 inch cooking tin, alternating between beef and cauliflower until both are gone. Dispense the egg mixture onto the meat and cauliflower. Cook for a half hour.

Prep Instructions:

Cut casserole into 6 slices. Add 1 slice per meal prep container. Either store in the refrigerator for up to five days, or put in the freezer for 1 month.

Beef Recipe 5: Bell Pepper Nacho Slices

Prep time: 15 minutes; **Cook time:** 25 minutes;
Serving Size: 2 bell peppers; **Serves:** 9;
Calories: 145; **Total Fat:** 9 g; **Protein:** 13 g;
Total Carbs: 4 g; **Net Carbs:** 3 g; **Sugar:** 2 g; **Fiber:** 1 g;

Ingredients:

- 1 pound lean ground beef
- 1 teaspoon cumin
- 1 teaspoon chili powder
- Pepper and salt, as necessary
- 3 bell peppers, cut into thick strips
- 1 cup Mexican cheese blend
- ¾ cup your favorite salsa

Directions:

Heat oven to 375 degrees Fahrenheit. Cook the ground beef on a skillet or a pan on the stove until brown. Mix the ground beef with the rest of the spices, and then mix in the salsa as well. Line the peppers on a cookie sheet and ladle a heap of ground beef mixture onto each one. Sprinkle cheese on top as well. Cook for ten minutes.

Prep Instructions:

Once the peppers are out of the oven, feel free to add any other toppings to these nachos, such as avocado, sour cream, or beans. Place bell peppers inside a storage container and refrigerate for up to 2-3 days.

Beef Recipe 6: Ketogenic Meatloaf

Prep time: 10 minutes; **Cook time:** 40 minutes;
Serving Size: 3 meatloaf slices; **Serves:** 6;
Calories: 383; **Total Fat:** 28.82 g; **Protein:** 23.98 g;
Total Carbs: 6.43 g; **Net Carbs:** 4.73 g; **Sugar:** 2.7 g; **Fiber:** 1.7 g;

Ingredients:

- 1 container of low-fat marinara sauce
- 1 pound of ground beef
- 1 teaspoon Worcestershire sauce
- 12 ounces of mushrooms, diced
- 1 tablespoon thyme
- 1 tablespoon oregano
- ¼ cup flour, almond
- 2 eggs
- 1 tablespoon tomato paste
- 2 minced garlic cloves
- ¼ cup unsweetened almond milk
- 1 onion, diced

Directions:

Heat oven to 350 degrees Fahrenheit. Mix all of the ingredients in a bowl, except for the pasta sauce. This will create your tasty meatloaf. In a bread pan, pack in the meatloaf blend. Ladle the pasta sauce over the meatloaf. Heat for 40 minutes, making sure that it is fully cooked through before cutting up.

Prep Instructions:

Do your best to make each slice of meatloaf be the same size. This way, you'll be able to have exactly 18 pieces, easily yielding 6 servings of meatloaf. Refrigerate for up to 4 days.

Beef Recipe 7: Skinny Blue Cheese Burgers

Prep time: 10 minutes; **Cook time:** 10 minutes;
Serving Size: 1 burger; **Serves:** 9;
Calories: 708; **Total Fat:** 59 g; **Protein:** 347 g;
Total Carbs: 3 g; **Net Carbs:** 2 g; **Sugar:** .5 g; **Fiber:** 1 g;

Ingredients:

- 3 pounds lean ground beef
- 12 ounces blue cheese crumbles
- 3 tablespoons steak spice
- 3 tablespoons Worcestershire sauce
- 9 Portobello mushrooms
- 18 ounces onion rounds

Directions:

To make the burger patties, combine the ground beef, blue cheese, the Worcestershire sauce, and the steak spice. Combine until well-mixed, and then assemble into 9 equal size patties. Next, cut your Portobello mushrooms so that the stems are removed and a beef patty could easily sit on top. Place the onions into a pan and cook until translucent, about two-three minutes. Finally, cook your burger patty in another pan on each side for about 10 minutes total.

Prep Instructions:

It's probably be best to assemble your burger when you're ready to eat it, rather than beforehand. Simply combine 1 Portobello mushroom, 1 beef patty, and 3 onion rounds. There is no need for a bread bun with this recipe. Refrigerate for up to 3 days.

Chicken Recipe 8: General Tso's Meatballs

Prep time: 10 minutes; **Cook time:** 20 minutes;
Serving Size: 4 meatballs; **Serves:** 8;
Calories: 322; **Total Fat:** 3.75 g; **Protein:** 23 g;
Total Carbs: 10.25 g; **Net Carbs:** 3.75 g; **Sugar:** 1 g; **Fiber:** 2 g;

Ingredients:

- 2 pounds ground chicken
- 2 eggs
- 6 tablespoons rice vinegar
- ½ cup flour, almond
- 2 teaspoons garlic powder
- 6 tablespoons soy sauce
- ½ cup minced scallions
- 4 tablespoons ginger
- 1 teaspoon sesame oil
- 6 tablespoons Stevia
- Cooking oil, as necessary
- ¼ cup water

Directions:

Combine the following ingredients in a mixing bowl: chicken, ginger, scallions, garlic powder, almond flour, and egg. Once these ingredients are combined well, create 32 small meatballs. Heat up a skillet, pour in the oil, and fry these balls until they're cooked through completely. In a separate bowl, mix the Stevia, rice vinegar, sesame oil, soy sauce and water. This will be the sauce for the meatballs. Once cooked, pour the sauce over all of the meatballs. Enjoy.

Prep Instructions:

Lay out 8 meal prep containers and place 4 meatballs into each one. Next, evenly distribute the sauce amongst all of the containers. Place meatballs inside refrigerator for up to 3 days.

Chicken Recipe 9: Chicken, Spinach & Feta Frittata

Prep time: 10 minutes; **Cook time:** 30 minutes;
Serving Size: 1/12 of the frittata; **Serves:** 12;
Calories: 206; **Total Fat:** 16 g; **Protein:** 12 g;
Total Carbs: 3 g; **Net Carbs:** 1.4 g; **Sugar:** 1 g; **Fiber:** 1.6 g;

Ingredients:

- 12 ounces raw chicken
- 10 ounces of spinach
- ¼ teaspoon nutmeg
- ½ teaspoon pepper
- ½ teaspoon salt
- ½ cup milk
- ½ cup whipping cream
- 12 eggs
- ½ cup feta

Directions:

Heat oven to 375 degrees Fahrenheit. Spray a pie pan with low-fat cooking spray. Set aside. Tear the chicken into little pieces and put into a mixing bowl. Make sure that the spinach is dry before tearing this as well and putting it into the same bowl as the chicken. Mix in the feta and combine. Pat this evenly into the pie pan. In another dish, mix together the spices, milk, whipping cream, and eggs. Once combined, pour this on top of the flat chicken layer. Cook in the oven for a half hour.

Prep Instructions:

Instead of cooking this recipe in a pie pan, you also have the option of cooking it in muffin tins. This recipe will yield 18 muffins, which might be preferable if you're looking to cook in an extremely large batch. Divide muffins among plastic bags and refrigerate for up to 3 days or freeze for up to 1 month.

Chicken Recipe 10: Super Simple Chicken Nuggets

Prep time: 15 minutes; **Cook time:** 10 minutes;
Serving Size: 4 nuggets; **Serves:** 8;
Calories: 196; **Total Fat:** 17 g; **Protein:** 9 g;
Total Carbs: 3 g; **Net Carbs:** 1 g; **Sugar:** 1 g; **Fiber:** 2 g;

Ingredients:

- 2 breasts of chicken
- 2 tablespoons oil
- ½ teaspoon salt, plus more for brining
- ½ teaspoon pepper
- 1 cup flour, almond
- 1 teaspoon vinegar, apple cider
- ¼ cup mayonnaise

Directions:

Heat oven to 450 degrees Fahrenheit. Place parchment paper on a cookie sheet and set aside. Pour water into a bowl, and put the breasts of chicken in it with a tablespoon of salt. Allow the chicken to brine for between ten minutes and 1 hour. Slice the chicken into nuggets. In a separate bowl, combine the flour with ½ teaspoon of salt and all of the pepper. Mix together the vinegar and mayonnaise. Take each nugget and dip it into the mayonnaise before coating it with almond flour. Place each nugget on the cookie pan. Cook on each side for 7 minutes.

Prep Instructions:

This recipe will leave you with 32 nuggets. Divide these into 8 servings by putting 4 nuggets into 8 meal prep containers. Refrigerate the nuggets for up to 3 days. Serve with a steamed vegetable such as broccoli.

Chicken Recipe 11: Refreshing Caprese Chicken

Prep time: 10 minutes; **Cook time:** 25 minutes; **Serving Size:** 1 chicken breast; **Serves:** 8; **Calories:** 365; **Total Fat:** 21 g; **Protein:** 39 g; **Total Carbs:** 4 g; **Net Carbs:** 3 g; **Sugar:** 1 g; **Fiber:** 1 g;

Ingredients:

- 4 chicken breasts, sliced half to make 8 pieces
- ½ cup basil
- 4 tablespoons olive oil
- 4 tablespoons balsamic vinegar
- 4 Roma tomatoes, cut into thick slices
- 8 ounces cheese, mozzarella
- Pepper and salt, as necessary

Directions:

Heat oven to 400 degrees Fahrenheit. Put parchment paper on a cookie pan. Set aside. Season each slice of chicken with salt and pepper. Place each slice of chicken onto the cookie sheet, before cutting up the tomatoes and mozzarella and topping each slice of chicken with it evenly. Next, pour the balsamic and oil over the chicken. Cook for 25 minutes. Garnish with basil.

Prep Instructions:

Simply place one slice of chicken into 8 a meal prep container of your choice and you're good to go. Store in the refrigerator for up to 5 days.

Chicken Recipe 12: Low Carb Chicken Parmesan

Prep time: 10 minutes; **Cook time:** 30 minutes;
Serving Size: 1 chicken breast; **Serves:** 8;
Calories: 600; **Total Fat:** 32 g; **Protein:** 74 g;
Total Carbs: 3 g; **Net Carbs:** 2.5 g; **Sugar:** 2 g; **Fiber:** .5 g;

Ingredients:

- 4 pounds chicken breast, sliced into 8 pieces
- 4 ounces pork rinds
- 4 ounces parmesan cheese
- 4 eggs
- 2 cups pasta sauce
- 2 cups mozzarella, shredded
- Salt, pepper garlic powder and oregano as necessary

Directions:

Heat oven to 350 degrees Fahrenheit. Mix the pork rinds and parmesan in a food processor. Allow this mixture to become coarse, but not wet. Set aside. Crack and whip your eggs into a bowl, and dip each chicken piece into it, before dipping it into the pork and parmesan breading. Place each chicken piece onto a lined cookie sheet. Cook for 20 minutes. When cooked, take out of the oven and pour the pasta sauce over each chicken slice. Also drizzle the mozzarella cheese over the chicken. Cook for an additional 10 minutes so that the cheese melts. Enjoy.

Prep Instructions:

Simply place into 8 meal prep containers. Enjoy within 1 week, or opt to store half of this recipe in the freezer for up to 1 month.

Chicken Recipe 13: Asparagus, Chicken & Bacon Plate

Prep time: 5 minutes; **Cook time:** 30 minutes;
Serving Size: 1 chicken breast and ½ cup of asparagus & bacon;
Serves: 8;
Calories: 439; **Total Fat:** 18.2 g; **Protein:** 63 g;
Total Carbs: 4 g; **Net Carbs:** 3 g; **Sugar:** 2 g; **Fiber:** 1 g;

Ingredients:

- 4 pounds chicken breast, sliced into 8 equal pieces
- 1 tablespoon avocado oil
- 1 pound asparagus
- 4 tomatoes, sundried and sliced into chunks
- 4 pieces of bacon, sliced into chunks
- 8 slices of swiss cheese

Directions:

Heat oven to 400 degrees Fahrenheit. Coat a cookie pan with oil by spreading it evenly with a paper towel. Place chicken & asparagus slices onto cookie sheet, along with the tomatoes and bacon. Cook for 30 minutes, checking on the chicken to make sure that it's not getting too dry. When cooked, remove from oven and place asparagus, tomatoes, and bacon on top of chicken. Place 1 slice of swiss cheese on each chicken, and cook for 2 additional minutes.

Prep Instructions:

Divide the asparagus, tomatoes, and bacon into eighths, and place into 8 meal containers with 1 slice of chicken. Store inside refrigerate for up to 3 days. When eating, microwave for two and a half minutes.

Chapter 6

Seafood Recipes That Are Low in Carbs

Seafood Recipe 1: Sardine Fish Patties

Prep time: 15 minutes; **Cook time:** 5 minutes;
Serving Size: 3 patties; **Serves:** 4;
Calories: 269; **Total Fat:** 23 g; **Protein:** 16 g;
Total Carbs: 4 g; **Net Carbs:** 1.8 g; **Sugar:** 1 g; **Fiber:** 2.2 g;

Ingredients:

- 6 ounces sardines
- 4 eggs
- 2 cups cilantro
- ½ teaspoon salt
- ½ cup flour, coconut
- 4 tablespoons coconut oil

Directions:

Begin by mashing the sardines with a fork in a bowl. In another bowl, mix together the eggs and salt. Next, mix in the cilantro and the mashed sardines. With this mixture, form 12 patties. Dip each patty into the flour. Heat up the oil, and heat each patty for about 2.5 minutes on each side. Dry the patties on a paper towel prior to storing.

Prep Instructions:

Wrap each patty in foil or plastic wrap. Keep inside refrigerator for up to 3 days. Heat up the patties in a microwave for 3-5 minutes before serving.

Seafood Recipe 2: Baked Shrimp with Garlic

Prep time: 10 minutes; **Cook time:** 10 minutes;
Serving Size: 2 shrimp kabobs; **Serves:** 12;
Calories: 400; **Total Fat:** 17 g; **Protein:** 43 g;
Total Carbs: 9 g; **Net Carbs:** 7 g; **Sugar:** 2 g; **Fiber:** 2 g;

Ingredients:

- 6 pounds peeled shrimp
- 3 chopped zucchinis
- 48 ounces minced garlic
- 12 mushrooms
- 9 tablespoons lemon juice
- 12 tablespoons ghee
- 9 teaspoons salt
- 12 diced bell peppers

Directions:

Heat oven to 400 degrees Fahrenheit. Mix together salt, garlic and ghee. Divide this mixture in half, so that half is used as sauce and half is used as dipping later. Skewer your vegetables and shrimp onto 24 skewers. On a cookie sheet, place as many skewers as will fit in an even layer. Each tray should cook for about 5 minutes, before being flipped and being cooked for an additional 5 minutes. Consume with more ghee sauce.

Prep Instructions:

Place two shrimp kabobs into six meal prep containers. Eat within four days, or store in the freezer for up to one month. Reheat for three minutes prior to serving.

Seafood Recipe 3: Tuna Poke with Avocado

Prep time: 10 minutes; **Cook time:** 0 minutes;
Serving Size: ¼ pound of ahi tuna mixture; **Serves:** 6;
Calories: 350; **Total Fat:** 20.1 g; **Protein:** 30.3 g;
Total Carbs: 9.5 g; **Net Carbs:** 3.9 g; **Sugar:** 2.5 g; **Fiber:** 5.6 g;

Ingredients:

- 1.5 pounds ahi tuna
- 3 tablespoons sesame oil
- 3 tablespoons garlic sauce
- 3 avocados
- 3 tablespoons sesame seeds
- 6 tablespoons soy sauce
- 6 scallions, diced

Directions:

Slice the tuna into bite-sized chunks. In a bowl, combine scallions, spices, oil, and soy sauce. Dip the tuna into this sauce until it's fully coated. Slice the avocados into bite-sized pieces as well, and then mix them into the tuna. Drizzle the sesame seeds on top.

Prep Instructions:

This recipe is going to taste best refrigerated. You should not allow this recipe to sit in the refrigerator for longer than 3 days, because you are consuming raw fish. Some people opt to consume poke with bread, but since you're trying to be low-carb you can instead use celery or some other crunchy vegetable for a nice dipping variation.

Seafood Recipe 4: Shrimp & Vegetable Medley Casserole

Prep time: 15 minutes; **Cook time:** 30 minutes; **Serving Size:** 1 slice of casserole; **Serves:** 6; **Calories:** 253; **Total Fat:** 17.1 g; **Protein:** 17.2 g; **Total Carbs:** 9.3 g; **Net Carbs:** 6.3 g; **Sugar:** 4.2 g; **Fiber:** 3 g;

Ingredients:

- 18 peeled shrimps
- 2 eggs
- 1 tomato, sliced into thick chunks
- 1 tablespoon butter
- 2.5 ounces minced garlic cloves
- 2 zucchinis, sliced into thick chunks
- ¼ cup yellow onion
- ½ cup cheese, parmesan
- ½ cup flour, almond
- ½ teaspoon salt
- 1/3 cup whipping cream
- ½ teaspoon pepper
- Cilantro as a topping

Directions:

Heat oven to 350 degrees Fahrenheit. Layer all of the vegetables into the base of a baking pan. Place shrimp on top of vegetables. In a mixing bowl, combine eggs, garlic, flour, whipping cream, butter and your spices. Pour this evenly over the entire casserole dish. Next, cook this casserole for a half hour.

Prep Instructions:

You'll know that this casserole is done when the top of it looks crispy. Slice into 6 equal pieces and store in meal prep containers. This will keep in the refrigerator for up to 1 week.

Seafood Recipe 5: Shrimp with Thai Curry Sauce

Prep time: 5 minutes; **Cook time:** 15 minutes;
Serving Size: 1 cup of curry with shrimp; **Serves:** 8;
Calories: 228; **Total Fat:** 9.6 g; **Protein:** 26.2 g;
Total Carbs: 8.7 g; **Net Carbs:** 6.7 g; **Sugar:** 5.2 g; **Fiber:** 2 g;

Ingredients:

- 2 pounds peeled shrimp
- 14 ounces snap peas
- 2 teaspoons olive oil
- 4 tablespoons fish sauce
- 2 minced garlic cloves
- 2 onions, diced
- 6 tablespoons curry paste
- 2 cans milk, coconut

Directions:

Start by cooking the oil and garlic on a skillet with oil. Cook until the onion is see-through, before adding the curry paste, fish sauce, and milk. Bring this mixture to a bubble, and let it cook for ten minutes. Place snap peas into milky sauce and cook for three minutes. Finally, mix in shrimp and heat for roughly 2 minutes.

Prep Instructions:

Depending on the size of your pan, you may want to cook this recipe in two separate batches. The shrimp will completely cook through and gain the flavor of the curry sauce more fully. The snap peas complement this meal nicely, so all you have to do is ladle 1 cup of the curry into 8 meal prep containers for a week's worth of lunch or dinner.

Seafood Recipe 6: Light Ceviche

Prep time: 10 minutes; **Cook time:** 0 minutes;
Serving Size: ½ pound of ceviche; **Serves:** 8;
Calories: 210; **Total Fat:** 2 g; **Protein:** 41 g;
Total Carbs: 6 g; **Net Carbs:** 3 g; **Sugar:** 1 g; **Fiber:** 3 g;

Ingredients:

- 4 pounds tilapia
- 8 ounces onion, diced
- 16 ounces diced cucumber
- 12 ounces tomato, diced
- ¼ cup lemon juice
- 4 serrano peppers
- 8 tablespoons cilantro
- ½ tablespoon salt

Directions:

Slice all of the tilapia into small chunks. Place into a bowl and combine with the remaining ingredients, except for the salt. Once combine, sprinkle the salt on top. Place inside refrigerator for up to 6 hours before serving.

Prep Instructions:

Since you're meal prepping and are probably not planning to consume this recipe as soon as you make it, this shouldn't be a problem. The acid from the lemon juice is able to "cook" the fish, so that it is technically still raw but has also been altered from a compositional perspective. Store in refrigerator for up to 1-2 days.

Seafood Recipe 7: Salmon Stuffed with Crab

Prep time: 10 minutes; **Cook time:** 25 minutes;
Serving Size: 4 ounces of salmon; **Serves:** 8;
Calories: 243; **Total Fat:** 13 g; **Protein:** 29 g;
Total Carbs: 1 g; **Net Carbs:** .8 g; **Sugar:** .5 g; **Fiber:** .2 g;

Ingredients:

- 2 pounds salmon fillet, cut into 8 pieces
- 2 minced garlic cloves
- 8 ounces crab meat
- 1 teaspoon old bay spice
- ½ onion, diced
- 2 tablespoons butter, melted
- 2 tablespoons parsley
- 2 1.5 tablespoons lemon juice
- 2 tablespoons mayonnaise

Directions:

Heat oven to 400 degrees Fahrenheit. Line a cookie pan with tin foil. Next, cook the onion on the stove until clear. In a bowl, combine mayonnaise, 1 tablespoon of lemon juice, parsley, garlic, and old bay. Beat the onion into this mixture. Mix in the crab. On the cookie sheet, place the fillets of salmon. In the middle of the salmon, fold in the crab filling. In yet another bowl, mix the butter with the remaining lemon juice. Pour this over each salmon fillet. Drizzle with salt and pepper as necessary. Cook for 18 minutes and garnish with parsley.

Prep Instructions:

Divide equal serving portions of the stuffed salmon into glass containers and keep inside the refrigerator for up to 3 days. Serve each meal with a side of kale or broccoli for a complete and incredibly satisfying meal.

Seafood Recipe 8: Crab and Avocado Quick Salad

Prep time: 10 minutes; **Cook time:** 0 minutes;
Serving Size: ½ avocado & 4 ounces of crab meat blend; **Serves:** 8;
Calories: 178; **Total Fat:** 13 g; **Protein:** 9.5 g;
Total Carbs: 9 g; **Net Carbs:** 4 g; **Sugar:** 1 g; **Fiber:** 5 g;

Ingredients:

- 4 avocados
- 4 tablespoons cilantro
- 4 tablespoons olive oil
- 16 ounces crab meat
- 2 tablespoons lime juice
- 8 tablespoons yellow onion
- 12 grape tomatoes, halved

Directions:

Start by halving the avocados and removing the pits. You can also remove the skin, so that you're only left with the avocado meat. In a bowl, combine the rest of the ingredients, making sure to coat the crab meat well. Finally, scoop the crab meat mixture into each avocado.

Prep Instructions:

For this recipe, it might make more sense to cut each avocado in half, but keep the skin of each avocado intact. Place half the avocado into a meal prep container, and ladle 4 ounces of the crab blend into the container separately. This way, the avocado won't brown, and you can scoop the crab into the avocado when you're ready to eat it. Refrigerate for up to 1 week.

Seafood Recipe 9: Flounder Wrapped in Foil

Prep time: 15 minutes; **Cook time:** 10 minutes;
Serving Size: 1 flounder filet; **Serves:** 8;
Calories: 194; **Total Fat:** 8 g; **Protein:** 27 g;
Total Carbs: 3 g; **Net Carbs:** 2 g; **Sugar:** 0 g; **Fiber:** 1 g;

Ingredients:

- 8 cod fillets
- 8 teaspoons olive oil
- 4 teaspoons parsley
- 8 thin slices of lemon
- 8 pieces tin foil

Directions:

Heat oven to 400 degrees Fahrenheit. Lay out 8 slices of tin foil. Place a cod fillet on top of each one. Sprinkle each fillet with 1 teaspoon of oil. Top with a slice of lemon and a ½ teaspoon parsley. Fold the tin foil so that the fish is completely wrapped. Bake for 20 minutes, until fish is flaky.

Prep Instructions:

For this recipe, as long as the fish are roughly the same size and you check to make sure that one is cooked through, there's little need to remove the fish from the foil until you're ready to eat it. Refrigerate for up to 3 days.

Seafood Recipe 10: Calamari Salad

Prep time: 5 minutes; **Cook time:** 15 minutes;
Serving Size: 1 cup; **Serves:** 8;
Calories: 121.6; **Total Fat:** 1.7 g; **Protein:** 18.3 g;
Total Carbs: 7.9 g; **Net Carbs:** 7 g; **Sugar:** 1.2 g; **Fiber:** 0.9 g;

Ingredients:

- 2 pounds squid
- 2 tablespoons red wine vinegar
- ½ cup parsley
- 1 cup roasted red peppers, sliced
- 2 minced garlic cloves
- ½ cup red onion, diced
- 1 cup celery, diced
- ½ juice of a lemon

Directions:

Slice the squid into ringlets and tentacle pieces that can be easily consumed. In the meantime, mix together the onion, peppers, lemon juice, vinegar, parsley, celery, and garlic. Place a pot on the stove filled with water and boil. Boil the calamari for roughly sixty seconds. Setup a bucket filled with ice water. After cooking the calamari, place the cooked calamari into this freezing water. Let the calamari sit in this ice for 5 minutes. Finally, combine the calamari with the onion and pepper mixture.

Prep Instructions:

Simply place 1 cup of the salad into 8 individual meal prep containers and refrigerate for 3-5 days.

Seafood Recipe 11: Roasted Red Snapper

Prep time: 10 minutes; **Cook time:** 20 minutes;
Serving Size: 6 ounces; **Serves:** 6;
Calories: 256.6; **Total Fat:** 6.1 g; **Protein:** 45.3 g;
Total Carbs: 3.2 g; **Net Carbs:** 3 g; **Sugar:** .3 g; **Fiber:** .2 g;

Ingredients:

- 6 red snapper fillets
- 1.5 tablespoons breadcrumbs
- 6 teaspoons olive oil
- 6 slices lemon
- 2 minced garlic cloves
- 3 tablespoons oregano

Directions:

Heat oven to 450 degrees Fahrenheit. Coat a cookie sheet with tin foil. Drizzle a teaspoon of oil onto each fillet. Once coated in oil, also douse each fillet with garlic and oregano. Coat one side of the fish with breadcrumbs, before placing on the cookie sheet. Cook for 20 minutes.

Prep Instructions:

Each filet can be served with a lemon wedge. Divide into equal portions among 6 storage containers. Freeze for up to 1 month, or consume refrigerated for up to 5 days.

Seafood Recipe 12: Baked Cod with Cheese

Prep time: 10 minutes; **Cook time:** 15 minutes; Serving Size: 1 filet of cod; **Serves:** 8; Calories: 247; **Total Fat:** 15 g; **Protein:** 20 g; Total Carbs: 7 g; **Net Carbs:** 7 g; Sugar: 2 g; Fiber: 0 g;

Ingredients:

- 8 slices of cod
- 2 teaspoons Worcestershire
- 1.5 cups mayonnaise
- 8 scallions, diced
- ½ cup pecorino Romano cheese

Directions:

Heat oven to 400 degrees Fahrenheit. Drizzle a dish with oil. Set aside. In a bowl, mix together mayonnaise, scallions, pecorino Romano, and Worcestershire. Place the cod into the dish and pour the mayonnaise mixture over it. Cook for 15 minutes, until the cod is nice and flaky.

Prep Instructions:

Place each fillet of cod in a meal prep container. Freeze for up to 1 month, or consume refrigerated for up to 3 days. Serve with a slice of lemon for an extra kick of zest.

Seafood Recipe 13: Dijon Mustard Salmon with Garlic & Herbs

Prep time: 20 minutes; **Cook time:** 20 minutes;
Serving Size: 1 slice of salmon; **Serves:** 8;
Calories: 233.5; **Total Fat:** 8 g; **Protein:** 35 g;
Total Carbs: 3 g; **Net Carbs:** 2.5 g; **Sugar:** .5 g; **Fiber:** .5 g;

Ingredients:

- 12 ounces of salmon, sliced into 8 equal pieces
- 4 tablespoons Dijon
- 2 teaspoons red wine vinegar
- 4 minced garlic cloves
- 2 teaspoons allspice
- 2 teaspoons oil
- 8 wedges of a lemon

Directions:

Combine the Dijon, garlic, allspice, oil and vinegar in a food processor. In a pan on the stove, cook each piece of salmon, seasoning with salt and pepper as you do so. Heat each side of the fish for about 6 minutes on medium heat. Ladle 1/8 of the Dijon sauce that you've already made into the pan with the fish, cooking each side to make sure that it's full of flavor. Serve with lemon wedges.

Prep Instructions:

Since Dijon mustard is not full of carbohydrates, it might be a good idea to make extra Dijon sauce for this recipe. This way, you can prep each salmon fillet to have extra sauce with it, without having to worry about the carbs that are involved. Divide the salmon among 8 storage containers and place inside refrigerator for up to 3 days.

Chapter 7
Healthy Soups for Slurping

Soup Recipe 1: Cauliflower Soup with Ham

Prep time: 15 minutes; **Cook time:** 35 minutes;
Serving Size: ½ cup of soup; **Serves:** 10;
Calories: 120; **Total Fat:** 10 g; **Protein:** 7.1 g;
Total Carbs: 11 g; **Net Carbs:** 6.9 g; **Sugar:** 2.7 g; **Fiber:** 4.1 g;

Ingredients:

- 6 cups cauliflower pieces
- 6 cups chicken broth
- 2 cups water
- ½ teaspoon of each: onion & garlic powder
- 3 cups ham, diced
- 2 tablespoons vinegar, apple cider
- 1 tablespoon thyme
- 2 tablespoons butter
- Pepper and salt as necessary

Directions:

In a soup pot, combine the cauliflower, chicken broth, and onion and garlic powder. Bring to boil, and then let this to bubble for about 25 minutes. Insert a hand blender into the soup pot and pulse until everything is blended nicely. Add the ham and thyme leaves. Cook for another 10 minutes. Finally, mix in the butter and vinegar. Add pepper and salt as needed.

Prep Instructions:

Simply place ½ cup of the soup into 10 meal prep soup containers and refrigerate. Eat within seven days, as the vinegar should be able to keep this recipe good for a bit longer than some of the other ones.

Soup Recipe 2: Low Carb Chicken Veggie Soup

Prep time: 15 minutes; **Cook time:** 15 minutes;
Serving Size: 1.5 cups; **Serves:** 6;
Calories: 310; **Total Fat:** 16 g; **Protein:** 34 g;
Total Carbs: 6 g; **Net Carbs:** 4 g; **Sugar:** 3 g; **Fiber:** 2 g;

Ingredients:

- 9 cups chicken broth
- 3 celery stalks, diced
- 3 peeled and diced zucchinis
- 3 breasts of chicken, cut into chunks
- 3 scallions, diced
- 6 tablespoons oil, avocado
- ½ cup cilantro
- Salt as necessary

Directions:

Place oil in a pan and cook with the chicken until the chicken's cooked. Mix in the broth and bring pan to a simmer. Add in scallions and celery. Finally, mix in the zucchini and cilantro. Allow to cook for ten additional minutes before removing from heat.

Prep Instructions:

You may have to cook this recipe in batches, since there is going to be a lot going into the stovetop pan. A nice garnish for this recipe would be ¼ cup cashews along with the 1.5 cups of soup. Keep in refrigerator for up to 3 days. Heat up the soup in a microwave for 3-5 minutes before serving.

Soup Recipe 3: Crème of Broccoli Soup

Prep time: 15 minutes; **Cook time:** 30 minutes;
Serving Size: 1 cup; **Serves:** 8;
Calories: 166; **Total Fat:** 6 g; **Protein:** 9.9 g;
Total Carbs: 23.5 g; **Net Carbs:** 15.5 g; **Sugar:** 9.9 g; **Fiber:** 8 g;

Ingredients:

- 16 cups broccoli pieces
- 2 onions, diced
- 2 tablespoons olive oil
- 2 stalks celery, diced
- 1 teaspoon of each: onion & garlic powder
- 8 cups cauliflower pieces
- 6 cups chicken broth
- 3 cups milk, almond & unsweetened
- 2 teaspoons salt
- ½ teaspoon pepper
- ¼ teaspoon celery seeds

Directions:

In a soup pan, heat oil. Place onion, celery, pepper & salt into the pot and cook until the onion is translucent. Mix in the garlic & onion powder, celery seeds, 6 cups broccoli, all of the cauliflower & the broth. Cook for 9 minutes. Once tender, transfer this soup to a blender. Pulse until smooth. Transfer back to the soup pot, and mix in the rest of the broccoli and milk. Bring to a bubble and cook for roughly 25 more minutes.

Prep Instructions:

Divide the soup among 4 glass containers and refrigerate for up to 3 days. Heat up the soup in a microwave for 3-5 minutes before serving.

Soup Recipe 4: Avocado and Mint Cold Soup

Prep time: 5 minutes; **Cook time:** 0 minutes;
Serving Size: ½ cup; **Serves:** 6;
Calories: 280; **Total Fat:** 26 g; **Protein:** 4 g;
Total Carbs: 12 g; **Net Carbs:** 4 g; **Sugar:** 2 g; **Fiber:** 8 g;

Ingredients:

- 3 avocados
- 6 leaves of romaine
- ¼ cup mint leaves
- 3 cups milk
- 3 tablespoons lime juice
- Salt as necessary

Directions:

Simply place all of these soup parts into a blender. Pulse until smooth.

Prep Instructions:

This soup is going to be better if it's refrigerated prior to consuming. Place ½ cup of the soup into 6 meal prep containers and refrigerate for up to 1 week.

Soup Recipe 5: Cauliflower & Garlic Soup

Prep time: 10 minutes; **Cook time:** 40 minutes;
Serving Size: 1 cup; **Serves:** 6;
Calories: 73; **Total Fat:** 2.4 g; **Protein:** 2.1 g;
Total Carbs: 11.3 g; **Net Carbs:** 9.2 g; **Sugar:** 4.1 g; **Fiber:** 2.1 g;

Ingredients:

- 2 bulbs of garlic
- 6 cups vegetable broth
- 5 cups cauliflower pieces
- ¾ teaspoon salt
- 1 tablespoon olive oil
- 3 chopped shallots

Directions:

Heat oven to 400 degrees Fahrenheit. Cut off the top of the garlic bulb and wrap each bulb in tin foil along with ½ teaspoon oil. Cook in the oven for a half hour. Place a pot on the stove and add in the rest of the oil. Cook the shallots for 5 minutes, before adding the garlic from the bulb. Add the remaining soup parts. Cook for about 12 minutes. In a blender, puree all of the ingredients.

Prep Instructions:

Simply place 1 cup of the soup into 6 meal prep containers. Keep in refrigerator for up to 5 days. Heat up the soup in a microwave for 3-5 minutes before serving.

Soup Recipe 6: Kale & Sausage Soup

Prep time: 10 minutes; **Cook time:** 20 minutes;
Serving Size: ½ cup; **Serves:** 6;
Calories: 300; **Total Fat:** 22.71 g; **Protein:** 16.31 g;
Total Carbs: 8.49 g; **Net Carbs:** 6.34 g; **Sugar:** 2 g; **Fiber:** 2.15 g;

Ingredients:

- 1 pound sausage
- 1 tablespoon butter
- 1 cup whipping cream
- ½ teaspoon chili powder
- 1 teaspoon of each: sage, basil, oregano
- 2 tablespoons red wine vinegar
- 2 minced garlic cloves
- 1 diced carrot
- 3 cups kale, sliced
- 4 cups chicken broth
- 1 diced yellow onion

Directions:

Heat up a soup pot, and place into it the sausage. Cook for 6 minutes. Remove from pan and pat to dry. In the pot, place the butter, onion and carrot. Cook until the onion is clear. Mix in garlic and vinegar, then the sage, chili powder, garlic, and basil. Bring to a simmer before adding cauliflower, kale and sausage. Cook for 15 minutes.

Prep Instructions:

Ladle a half cup of soup into 6 meal prep containers. Freezing this soup would be a good idea after a week of non-consumption. Heat up the soup in a microwave for 3-5 minutes before serving.

Soup Recipe 7: Bacon & Cheeseburger Soup

Prep time: 15 minutes; **Cook time:** 20 minutes;
Serving Size: ½ cup soup; **Serves:** 12;
Calories: 433; **Total Fat:** 35 g; **Protein:** 25.7 g;
Total Carbs: 3.8 g; **Net Carbs:** 3.2 g; **Sugar:** 1.5 g; **Fiber:** .6 g;

Ingredients:

- 24 ounces ground beef
- 6 ounces cream cheese
- 6 cups beef broth
- 1 teaspoon of each: garlic & onion powder, pepper and red pepper
- 10 bacon strips
- 4 tablespoons butter
- 5 tablespoons tomato paste
- 2 teaspoons of each: chili powder & cumin
- 6 diced dill pickles
- 4 teaspoons mustard
- 2 cups cheese, shredded
- 1 cup whipping cream

Directions:

In a pan, cook the bacon. Once cooked, remove from heat, but keep the bacon pan on the stove. Insert the ground beef into the pan with the bacon grease. In another pan, combine the butter with the rest of the spices on the list. Add in the cream cheese, mustard, shredded cheese, tomato paste & broth into the pan with the butter. Bake for 5 minutes. Finally, add in pickles and the whipping cream. Ladle this mixture over the ground beef. Bring to a bubble and bake for 10 minutes.

Prep Instructions:

This delicious recipe will leave you craving this soup for weeks. For more of a satisfying (yet more caloric) meal, consider using 6 meal prep containers and simply portioning 1 cup of soup into each one. Keep in refrigerator for up to 3 days. Heat up the soup in a microwave for 3-5 minutes before serving.

Soup Recipe 8: Simple Tomato Soup

Prep time: 5 minutes; **Cook time:** 2 minutes;
Serving Size: 1 cup; **Serves:** 8;
Calories: 187; **Total Fat:** 15.9 g; **Protein:** 3.5 g;
Total Carbs: 11.8 g; **Net Carbs:** 7.7 g; **Sugar:** 3.4 g; **Fiber:** 4.1 g;

Ingredients:

- 8 cups water
- 8 Roma tomatoes, cut into chunks
- 1 cup macadamia nuts, raw
- 2 minced garlic cloves
- ½ teaspoon basil
- 2 teaspoons salt
- 1 cup sun dried tomatoes

Directions:

This recipe is pretty simple. Place all of these soup parts into a blender and pulse for 5 minutes.

Prep Instructions:

You'll likely need to work these ingredients into a blender in batches. Perhaps dividing your ingredients into two and then blending is the way to go so that you don't end up losing the integrity of the recipe along the way. Keep in refrigerator for up to 5 days.

Soup Recipe 9: Mean Green Power Soup

Prep time: 5 minutes; **Cook time:** 2 minutes;
Serving Size: 1 cup of soup; **Serves:** 8;
Calories: 95; **Total Fat:** 7.6 g; **Protein:** 2.1 g;
Total Carbs: 6.7 g; **Net Carbs:** 2.5 g; **Sugar:** 1.1 g; **Fiber:** 4.2 g;

Ingredients:

- 2 avocados
- 2 minced garlic cloves
- 1 cup cucumber
- 2 tablespoons soy sauce
- 1 cup bell pepper, diced
- 4 leaves of spinach
- 2 scallions, diced
- ½ cup vegetable broth
- 2 tablespoons lemon juice
- Pepper and salt as necessary

Directions:

Put all of these fixings into a blender. Pulse until you're left with a soup-like consistency.

Prep Instructions:

While this soup can certainly be consumed in the evening, it could also serve well as a morning soup-smoothie of sorts. For meal prepping purposes, place 1 cup of soup into 8 separate containers. Keep in refrigerator for up to 5 days.

Soup Recipe 10: Gazpacho

Prep time: 10 minutes; **Cook time:** 10 minutes;
Serving Size: 1 cup of soup; **Serves:** 6;
Calories: 147; **Total Fat:** 9 g; **Protein:** 2.9 g;
Total Carbs: 16 g; **Net Carbs:** 13.4 g; **Sugar:** 8 g; **Fiber:** 2.6 g;

Ingredients:

- 1 chopped red onion
- 3 chopped tomatoes
- ½ chopped cucumber
- ½ chopped bell pepper
- 6 chopped celery stalks
- 1 minced garlic clove
- 3.5 cups tomato juice
- ¼ cup olive oil
- ¼ cup white vinegar
- ¼ cup parsley
- 1/8 teaspoon stevia

Directions:

In a food processor, combine the onion, tomatoes, cucumber, bell pepper, and celery stalks. Mix in the rest of the ingredients, and refrigerate prior to serving.

Prep Instructions:

Ladle 1 cup of soup into 6 meal prep containers. Allow to sit in the refrigerator for at least 3 hours prior to consuming. Keep in refrigerator for up to 5 days.

Soup Recipe 11: Chicken Stew & Vegetable Gumbo

Prep time: 10 minutes; **Cook time:** 45 minutes;
Serving Size: 1.5 cups of soup; **Serves:** 4;
Calories: 194; **Total Fat:** 2.9 g; **Protein:** 22.8 g;
Total Carbs: 19 g; **Net Carbs:** 14.5 g; **Sugar:** 6.9 g; **Fiber:** 4.5 g;

Ingredients:

- 4 chicken breasts, cut into chunks
- 1 yellow onion, diced
- 1 bell pepper, diced
- ½ teaspoon of each: mustard seed, oregano, salt
- ¼ teaspoon of each: turmeric, chili powder, pepper
- 2 cups kale, diced
- 2 garlic cloves, minced
- 2 teaspoons cumin
- 2 carrots, diced
- 1 rutabaga, cut into chunks

Directions:

In a slow cooker, combine the chicken, rutabaga, carrots, kale, onion, and bell pepper. In a bowl, mix together the rest of the soup parts. Mix this into the slow cooker. Cook for at least 45 minutes. If you have more time, allow this to cook even longer so that the vegetables became nice and soft.

Prep Instructions:

For this recipe, the longer that you cook the soup, the better; however, you can simply cook it for 45 minutes and then remember to microwave it when you're ready to eat it later in the week. Refrigerate for up to 5 days or freeze for up to a month. Heat up the soup in a microwave for 3-5 minutes before serving.

Soup Recipe 12: Italian Sausage Soup

Prep time: 10 minutes; **Cook time:** 20 minutes;
Serving Size: 2/3 cup of soup; **Serves:** 6;
Calories: 479; **Total Fat:** 43.8 g; **Protein:** 16 g;
Total Carbs: 6 g; **Net Carbs:** 4 g; **Sugar:** 1 g; **Fiber:** 2 g;

Ingredients:

- 16 ounces sausage
- 4 cups chicken broth
- 6 bacon slices
- 1 cup whipping cream
- 10 ounces spinach
- ½ diced yellow onion
- 2 minced garlic cloves

Directions:

Cook the sausage and the bacon together in a pan completely. Once cooked, mix in the garlic and onion. Combine in the spinach and broth. Cook until the spinach becomes wilted and the onions are fully cooked. Cook for an additional 15 minutes before adding the whipping cream.

Prep Instructions:

Divide the soup into glass storage containers. Keep in refrigerator for up to 3 days or freeze for up to a month. Heat up the soup in a microwave for 3-5 minutes before serving.

Soup Recipe 13: Chicken & Buffalo Soup

Prep time: 20 minutes; **Cook time:** 20 minutes; **Serving Size:** ¼ cup of soup **Serves:** 8; **Calories:** 564; **Total Fat:** 32.5 g; **Protein:** 57 g; **Total Carbs:** 4 g; **Net Carbs:** 3 g; **Sugar:** 1 g; **Fiber:** 1 g;

Ingredients:

- 8 breasts of chicken, cut into chunks
- 8 celery stalks, diced
- 1 teaspoon chili powder
- 4 carrots, diced
- 1 teaspoon thyme
- 1 cup whipping cream
- 4 ounces cream cheese
- 64 ounces chicken broth
- 1 cup hot sauce
- 2 tablespoons salt
- 12 tablespoons butter

Directions:

Place celery and carrots into a soup pan. Add chicken with some olive oil. Cover and let chicken cook through. Remove the chicken once it's done cooking, and then add the broth to the pot. Add in the butter, cream cheese, and whipping cream. Bring to a boil. Shred chicken into pieces and then place back into pot. Add the hot sauce and the rest of your spices.

Prep Instructions:

This soup goes well with scallion as a garnish, or with extra cheese on top if you don't mind additional calories. Refrigerate this soup for up to 3 days. Heat up the soup in a microwave for 3-5 minutes before serving.

Chapter 8
Salads Recipes So Good You'll Forget You're Eating One

Salad Recipe 1: Bacon, Avocado, & Chicken Breast Salad

Prep time: 5 minutes; **Cook time:** 15 minutes;
Serving Size: 3.5 ounces of chicken, 1 egg & ½ cup of salad mix;
Serves: 6;
Calories: 670; **Total Fat:** 48 g; **Protein:** 50 g;
Total Carbs: 12 g; **Net Carbs:** 5 g; **Sugar:** 1 g; **Fiber:** 7 g;

Ingredients:

- 3 avocados
- 21 ounces chicken breast
- 6 tablespoons vinegar, apple cider
- 6 ounces shredded cheese
- 6 hardboiled eggs
- 6 romaine lettuce heads
- 6 tablespoons olive oil
- 6 bacon strips

Directions:

Slice up the romaine into edible-size pieces. Cook up the chicken on the stove with some oil, along with the bacon. Chop up the bacon and the chicken into chunks, and then mix the rest of the ingredients with the romaine. Drizzle with olive oil as needed.

Prep Instructions:

This healthy, yet fueling, salad will keep your hunger pangs satisfied for a week. Divide equal amounts of salad into 6 meal prep containers and place inside refrigerator for up to 3 days.

Salad Recipe 2: Sophie Salad with Berries & Chicken

Prep time: 10 minutes; **Cook time:** 15 minutes;
Serving Size: ½ chicken breast and ½ cup salad mix; **Serves:** 8;
Calories: 338; **Total Fat:** 20 g; **Protein:** 22 g;
Total Carbs: 15 g; **Net Carbs:** 10 g; **Sugar:** 4 g; **Fiber:** 5 g;

Ingredients:

- 4 breasts of chicken, cut into chunks
- 12 tablespoons feta
- 3 cups blueberries
- 24 strawberries, sliced into small pieces
- 2 cups chopped walnuts
- 8 cups spinach
- 12 tablespoons raspberry balsamic vinegar

Directions:

Cook the chicken chunks in a pan until fully cooked, about fifteen minutes. Take away from heat and permit to cool. In the meantime, combine the rest of your ingredients into a bowl. Top with the chicken chunks and your vinegar dressing.

Prep Instructions:

You can also opt to spice up this recipe with some avocado slices, some tomato, or some diced onion. Divide equal amounts of salad into 8 meal prep containers and place inside refrigerator for up to 3 days.

Salad Recipe 3: Low Carb Cobb Salad

Prep time: 10 minutes; **Cook time:** 10 minutes;
Serving Size: 1 cup of lettuce mix, 2 bacon strips & 1 egg; **Serves:** 6;
Calories: 605; **Total Fat:** 50 g; **Protein:** 45 g;
Total Carbs: 9 g; **Net Carbs:** 3 g; **Sugar:** 2 g; **Fiber:** 3 g;

Ingredients:

- 3 tablespoons white vinegar
- 1.5 avocado
- 12 bacon slices
- 12 ounces breast of chicken, cut into chunks
- 3 diced tomatoes
- 6 eggs hardboiled
- 6 cups spinach
- 6 tablespoons olive oil

Directions:

Start by cooking the chicken and bacon. While that's cooking, combined the rest of the ingredients, making sure that everything is bite-sized. Next, mix the salad parts with oil and vinegar. Finally, add the chicken and bacon. Mix well one more time.

Prep Instructions:

Each meal prep container should receive 1 cup of the lettuce mixture, making sure that each container has what looks to be 2 bacon strips and 1 egg. Place inside refrigerator for up to 3 days.

Salad Recipe 4: Mixed Green Salad

Prep time: 10 minutes; **Cook time:** 15 minutes;
Serving Size: 2 ounces of salad, 2 bacon slices; **Serves:** 6;
Calories: 480; **Total Fat:** 38 g; **Protein:** 17.5 g;
Total Carbs: 10 g; **Net Carbs:** 4.3 g; **Sugar:** 5 g; **Fiber:** 6.7 g;

Ingredients:

- 12 bacon slices
- 18 tablespoons pine nuts
- 12 tablespoons grated parmesan
- 12 ounces lettuce
- 12 tablespoons raspberry balsamic dressing
- Pepper and salt as necessary

Directions:

Cook bacon and then rip into small pieces. Mix the rest of the salad parts, mixing in the bacon last. Drizzle the dressing over the salad. Serve chilled.

Prep Instructions:

Instead of drizzling the dressing on the salad beforehand, it might be a better idea to put the dressing into dressing meal prep containers. This will prevent salad sogginess. Refrigerate salad for up to 3 days.

Salad Recipe 5: Bacon & Brussels Sprouts Salad

Prep time: 5 minutes; **Cook time:** 30 minutes;
Serving Size: ¼ pound of Brussel sprouts; **Serves:** 8;
Calories: 280; **Total Fat:** 20 g; **Protein:** 13 g;
Total Carbs: 4 g; **Net Carbs:** 2.5 g; **Sugar:** 2 g; **Fiber:** 1.5 g;

Ingredients:

- 4 tablespoons olive oil
- 2 pounds Brussels sprouts
- 16 slices of bacon
- Pepper and salt as necessary

Directions:

Heat oven to 375 degrees Fahrenheit. Quarter all of the Brussels so that they're in nice, bite-sized pieces. Season with pepper, oil and salt. Place on a cookie pan, and bake for a half hour, flipping them over halfway. Cook the bacon on the stovetop, and rip into small pieces. Once the Brussels are finished cooking, combine them with the bacon.

Prep Instructions:

This recipe should keep well in the refrigerator for about a week. Either eat cold, or microwave before consuming. Each meal prep container should receive ¼ pound of Brussels sprouts.

Salad Recipe 6: Mozzarella, Tomato & Basil Salad

Prep time: 5 minutes; **Cook time:** 0 minutes;
Serving Size: ½ tomato, ¼ lbs of mozzarella, & ½ tbs olive oil;
Serves: 8;
Calories: 190; **Total Fat:** 13 g; **Protein:** 10 g;
Total Carbs: 10 g; **Net Carbs:** 7 g; **Sugar:** 4 g; **Fiber:** 3 g;

Ingredients:

- 2 pounds mozzarella, cut into slices
- 4 tablespoons balsamic
- ¼ cup basil
- 4 tomatoes, cut into slices
- 4 tablespoons olive oil
- Pepper and salt as necessary

Directions:

Alternate the cheese and tomatoes on a plate or a tray. Pour the olive oil and balsamic on top, so that each slice of tomato and cheese is coated evenly. Garnish with basil.

Prep Instructions:

Instead of keeping the cheese and tomatoes in thick slices, you also have the option of chopping up the tomato and cheese and then mixing the oil and balsamic into it. This will keep in the refrigerator for up to five days. It's not recommended that you freeze this recipe.

Salad Recipe 7: Steak Salad with Balsamic & Veggies

Prep time: 15 minutes; **Cook time:** 25 minutes;
Serving Size: 0.4 ounces of steak, ½ cup vegetables; **Serves:** 8;
Calories: 450; **Total Fat:** 25 g; **Protein:** 32 g;
Total Carbs: 15 g; **Net Carbs:** 10 g; **Sugar:** 4 g; **Fiber:** 5 g;

Ingredients:

- 3 pounds sirloin steak
- 4 minced garlic cloves
- ½ cup balsamic vinegar
- 6 ounces sun dried tomatoes
- 6 tablespoons olive oil
- 8 ounces sliced mushrooms
- 2 sliced avocados
- 2 romaine lettuce heads
- 2 diced bell peppers
- 1 teaspoon of each: red pepper, Italian spice, onion powder, and garlic salt

Directions:

Slice all of the steak into thin strips. In a bowl, cover the steak with balsamic vinegar. Next, heat oil on a pan on the stove. Cook the onions, garlic, and mushrooms. These vegetables should cook for around 20 minutes. While that's happening, place the steak strips on a broiling pan. Season with your 1 teaspoon of spices. Broil for 6 minutes. Take away from heat, then combine with the rest of your salad parts.

Prep Instructions:

Be sure that your meal prep containers for this salad have separate compartments. This way, the lettuce will not wilt. Divide equal portions among storage containers and refrigerate for up to 3 days.

Salad Recipe 8: Easy Keto Caesar Salad

Prep time: 15 minutes; **Cook time:** 15 minutes;
Serving Size: ½ cup lettuce, 1 anchovy, & 1 tbs cheese; **Serves:** 8;
Calories: 730; **Total Fat:** 40 g; **Protein:** 11 g;
Total Carbs: 16 g; **Net Carbs:** 1.8 g; **Sugar:** 3.2 g; **Fiber:** 14.2 g;

Ingredients:

- 2 yolks from an egg
- 8 anchovies
- 4 minced garlic cloves
- 8 tablespoons shaved parmesan, and more for garnish
- 16 tablespoons avocado oil
- 6 tablespoons vinegar, apple cider
- 2 teaspoons Dijon mustard
- 28 romaine lettuce leaves
- 4 ounces pork rinds

Directions:

In a blender, mix yolk, vinegar, and mustard. While the blender is going, pour in the oil gradually. Pulse until smooth. This should look almost like a mayonnaise. Remove from blender, and combine with anchovies, cheese, and garlic. Blend again until smooth. Combine with pork rinds, lettuce leaves, and extra cheese.

Prep Instructions:

The best option here is to make the dressing ahead of time and then use it as you eat the salad to avoid salad sogginess. Store this salad in glass containers and keep in refrigerator for up to 3 days.

Salad Recipe 9: Stuffed Avocado Salad

Prep time: 5 minutes; **Cook time:** 5 minutes;
Serving Size: 1 stuffed avocado; **Serves:** 6;
Calories: 120; **Total Fat:** 50 g; **Protein:** 28 g;
Total Carbs: 20 g; **Net Carbs:** 5.6 g; **Sugar:** 2 g; **Fiber:** 14.4 g;

Ingredients:

- 3 avocados
- 19.2 ounces sardines
- 6 tablespoons lemon juice
- 2 teaspoons turmeric
- 6 tablespoons mayonnaise
- 6 scallions
- 2 teaspoons salt

Directions:

Slice and de-pit the avocados, so that you're left with 6 avocado halves. Mash the sardines until they're ground, and then add to the sardines, scallions, turmeric, and mayonnaise. Mix well together. Scoop the meat from the avocados into the bowl with the sardines, so that you're only left with the avocado shells. Mash and mix in the avocado meat into the sardine mixture. Add in lemon juice and salt. Scoop the final mixture into the avocado shells.

Prep Instructions:

Instead of using meal prep containers for this recipe, you can opt to simply wrap each avocado portion in tin foil for easier transport and faster prep. This recipe can be refrigerated for up to 3 days.

Salad Recipe 10: Pesto Salad with Chicken

Prep time: 10 minutes; **Cook time:** 20 minutes;
Serving Size: ¼ lbs of chicken, 2 bacon slices, & ¼ cup salad;
Serves: 8;
Calories: 380; **Total Fat:** 28 g; **Protein:** 28 g;
Total Carbs: 9 g; **Net Carbs:** 3 g; **Sugar:** 2 g; **Fiber:** 6 g;

Ingredients:

- 2 pounds chicken, cut into chunks
- ½ cup mayonnaise
- 2 tablespoons pesto
- 12 bacon strips
- 2 avocados, diced
- 20 grape tomatoes, halved
- Lettuce leaves as needed

Directions:

Heat oven to 400 degrees Fahrenheit. Bake the chicken chunks for about 15 minutes. While that's cooking, cook the bacon on the stovetop until crisp. Remove the chicken chunks from heat and combine with bacon, avocado, tomatoes, pesto and mayonnaise.

Prep Instructions:

Divide equally among 8 meal prep containers and refrigerate for up to 3 days.

Salad Recipe 11: Perfect Greek Salad

Prep time: 10 minutes; **Cook time:** 10 minutes;
Serving Size: ½ cup salad mixture; **Serves:** 8;
Calories: 180; **Total Fat:** 28 g; **Protein:** 10 g;
Total Carbs: 12 g; **Net Carbs:** 8.5 g; **Sugar:** 2.7 g; **Fiber:** 3.5 g;

Ingredients:

- 8 tomatoes, cubed
- 8 tablespoons capers
- 14.2 ounces feta cheese
- 2 teaspoons oregano
- 8 tablespoons olive oil
- 2 cucumbers, diced
- 2 bell peppers, diced
- 2 red onions, diced
- 32 olives

Directions:

Put all the vegetables into a bowl, and then add the oregano, olives, and capers. Throw in the feta and oil. Toss to coat.

Prep Instructions:

Because there are no leaves in this recipe, it should be fine to coat the vegetables with olive oil, with no need to worry about potential sogginess. Place ½ cup of the salad mixture into 8 meal prep containers. Keep in refrigerator for no more than 3 days.

Salad Recipe 12: Avocado & Bacon Summer Salad

Prep time: 10 minutes; **Cook time:** 20 minutes;
Serving Size: 1 avocado, 2 slices of bacon, and 1 cup salad mix;
Serves: 8;
Calories: 220; **Total Fat:** 66 g; **Protein:** 15 g;
Total Carbs: 23 g; **Net Carbs:** 6.7 g; **Sugar:** 5 g; **Fiber:** 16.3 g;

Ingredients:

- 2 scallions
- 16 bacon strips
- 4 hardboiled eggs
- 8 avocados
- 2 lettuce heads
- 4 cups spinach

Directions:

Cook the bacon and then rip into small pieces. Slice the avocados into thin strips, and then place all of the salad parts together in a bowl. Drizzle with olive oil as needed.

Prep Instructions:

Each meal prep container should receive 1 avocado, 2 bacon strips, and 1 cup of spinach and lettuce combination. Divide this salad into 8 meal prep containers and keep inside refrigerator for up to 3 days.

Salad Recipe 13: Blueberry Lemon & Chicken Salad

Prep time: 10 minutes; **Cook time:** 10 minutes; **Serving Size:** 2 cups salad; **Serves:** 8; **Calories:** 500; **Total Fat:** 40 g; **Protein:** 28 g; **Total Carbs:** 5 g; **Net Carbs:** 1 g; **Sugar:** 3 g; **Fiber:** 4 g;

Ingredients:

- 2 cups blueberries
- 16 teaspoons lemon juice
- 4 pounds chicken, sliced into chunks
- 16 tablespoons oil, coconut
- 2 cups red onion, diced
- 35.3 ounces lettuce
- 16 tablespoons olive oil

Directions:

On the stovetop, cook the chicken chunks with the coconut oil. When finished, combine the chicken with the blueberries, onions, lettuce, olive oil and lemon juice. Enjoy.

Prep Instructions:

This salad is best when consumed after being refrigerated. Place 2 cups of salad into 8 meal prep containers. This salad will stay fresh inside the refrigerator for up to 3 days.

Chapter 9
Vegan Dishes for the Compassionate Heart

Vegan Recipe 1: Vegan "Fish" Tacos

Prep time: 10 minutes; **Cook time:** 20 minutes;
Serving Size: 1 avocado, 2 slices of bacon, and 1 cup salad mix;
Serves: 8;
Calories: 220; **Total Fat:** 66 g; **Protein:** 15 g;
Total Carbs: 23 g; **Net Carbs:** 6.7 g; **Sugar:** 5 g; **Fiber:** 16.3 g;

Ingredients:

- 6 tablespoons soy sauce
- 1.5 teaspoons garlic powder
- 1 tablespoon sesame oil
- 12 romaine lettuce leaves
- Lime juice as needed
- 3 cups hempseeds
- ¾ cups lemon juice
- ¾ cup water
- 3 cans hearts of palm, chopped and drained
- 1.5 teaspoons sriracha

Directions:

In a blender, process the hempseed, lemon juice, and water. Please note that you are looking for a cream-cheese like consistency. You may need to add more water in order to achieve this. Next, box together the sriracha, garlic powder, soy sauce, and hearts of palm. In a pan on the stovetop, cook the hearts of palm mixture in the sesame oil for 5 minutes. Finally, take the romaine lettuce leaves and line them up in a row. Spread the fish taco mix evenly over each piece of lettuce, garnishing with lime juice if desired.

Prep Instructions:

Each meal prep container should receive 2 lettuce tacos. Place the lettuce leaves on top of the taco filling, so that they don't become soggy and unusable. You can also wrap the lettuce in a paper towel, if you're really worried about the leaves becoming soggy while they're sitting in the refrigerator, waiting to be consumed.

Vegan Recipe 2: Makeshift Lox on Toast

Prep time: 5 minutes; **Cook time:** 30 minutes;
Serving Size: 1 cracker; **Serves:** 8;
Calories: 50; **Total Fat:** 3.5 g; **Protein:** .7 g;
Total Carbs: 5 g; **Net Carbs:** 2.5 g; **Sugar:** 3 g; **Fiber:** 2.5 g;

Ingredients:

- 1 teaspoon kelp flakes
- 2 tablespoons olive oil
- ½ teaspoon Himalayan salt
- 8 long rice crackers
- 4 large carrots, peeled and sliced thin
- 1 tablespoon tamari

Directions:

Heat oven to 375 degrees Fahrenheit. In a bowl, mix together, kelp flakes, tamari, salt, and olive oil. Add in the carrots and whisk together so that they become marinated. On a cookie sheet, place the coated carrots onto it and cook for a half hour. Allow to cool. Place on the crackers. Enjoy.

Prep Instructions:

Place crackers inside a glass storage container and keep inside refrigerator for up to 5 days.

Vegan Recipe 3: Cauliflower Jambalaya

Prep time: 20 minutes; **Cook time:** 20 minutes;
Serving Size: 1 cup; **Serves:** 8;
Calories: 105; Total Fat: 7.5 g; Protein: 3.5 g;
Total Carbs: 9 g; Net Carbs: 4.6 g; **Sugar:** 2 g; Fiber: 4.4 g;

Ingredients:

- 1 teaspoon onion powder
- Basil for garnish
- 6 cups cauliflower, riced
- 1.5 cups coconut milk
- 4 teaspoons sriracha

Directions:

Place all of the ingredients into a stovetop pan. Cook, covered for about 10 minutes. Lower the heat, and continue to cook for an additional ten minutes, until most of the milk has become absorbed. Garnish with basil.

Prep Instructions:

If you own a rice cooker, you have the simple option of cooking the cauliflower in that instead of a traditional stovetop pan. Place equal amounts of this recipe inside meal prep containers and store for up to 5 days.

Vegan Recipe 4: Onion Keto Pancakes

Prep time: 10 minutes; **Cook time:** 40 minutes;
Serving Size: 1 pancake; **Serves:** 8;
Calories: 200; **Total Fat:** 17 g; **Protein:** 3.3 g;
Total Carbs: 10 g; **Net Carbs:** 4.7 g; **Sugar:** 2.5 g; **Fiber:** 5.3 g;

Ingredients:

- 8 tablespoons tamari
- 8 teaspoons rice wine vinegar
- 8 minced garlic cloves
- 4 cups flour, coconut
- 4 teaspoons garlic powder
- 1 teaspoon salt
- 16 scallions, diced
- 2 cups sesame oil
- 8 cups water, plus 8 additional tablespoons

Directions:

In a bowl, blend all of the water, scallions, tamari and garlic together. Let this mixture sit for five minutes, and then combine with coconut flour. Roll out 8 balls from this dough. Heat up a skillet with the sesame oil, and flatten each dough ball on the skillet as it cooks. Cook each pancake for about 5 minutes on each side.

Prep Instructions:

A pro tip for this recipe is to create the dough balls prior to heating the skillet to cook. Wrap dough balls or final pancakes in foil or plastic wrap. These are best refrigerated for up to 4 days.

Vegan Recipe 5: Vegan Keto Vegetable Lettuce Wrap

Prep time: 5 minutes; **Cook time:** 10 minutes;
Serving Size: 1 lettuce wrap; **Serves:** 4;
Calories: 130; **Total Fat:** 9 g; **Protein:** 5 g;
Total Carbs: 10 g; **Net Carbs:** 6.5 g; **Sugar:** 3 g; **Fiber:** 3.5 g;

Ingredients:

- 1 cup carrots, sliced into thin strips
- 8 tablespoons sauerkraut
- 8 tablespoons tahini
- 4 large lettuce leaves

Directions:

Simple wash the leaves of lettuce and then place ¼ cup of carrots, 2 tablespoons sauerkraut, and 2 tablespoons tahini into each wrap.

Prep Instructions:

Instead of coating the leaves with the tahini, you can also opt to use the sauce as a dip, which might make things easier from a meal prep perspective. Place all wraps inside a meal prep container and keep inside fridge for up to 5 days.

Vegan Recipe 6: Quick Greek Flatbread

Prep time: 15 minutes; **Cook time:** 0 minutes;
Serving Size: 1 flatbread; **Serves:** 6;
Calories: 220; **Total Fat:** 19 g; **Protein:** 6.8 g;
Total Carbs: 10 g; **Net Carbs:** 4.8 g; **Sugar:** 2 g; **Fiber:** 5.2 g;

Ingredients:

- 6 rice crackers
- ¼ cup parsley
- ¼ cup dill
- 1 teaspoon lemon juice
- 1 tablespoon olive oil
- ½ cup olives, diced
- ¼ cup sun dried tomatoes, diced
- 2 scallions, diced

Directions:

In a bowl combine all of your ingredients. Simply place ¼ cup of the mixture onto the rice crackers, and enjoy these makeshift flatbreads.

Prep Instructions:

Add avocados to this recipe for a healthy fat that will help to round off the meal nicely. Store this recipe inside meal prep containers. Refrigerate for up to 5 days.

Vegan Recipe 7: Eggplant Lasagna

Prep time: 30 minutes; **Cook time:** 30 minutes; **Serving Size:** ¼ slice of eggplant lasagna; **Serves:** 4; **Calories:** 145; **Total Fat:** 10 g; **Protein:** 7 g; **Total Carbs:** 15 g; **Net Carbs:** 9 g; **Sugar:** 4 g; **Fiber:** 6 g;

Ingredients:

- 1 cup pasta sauce
- ½ cup mozzarella cheese
- 1 eggplant, sliced into thin rounds
- 1 tablespoon salt
- 1 cup ricotta cheese
- 1 tablespoon olive oil

Directions:

Heat the oven to 375 degrees Fahrenheit. Prepare the eggplant by laying it out in a single layer and coating it with salt. Allow to dry out for about a half hour. Once it's dried out, clean the salt from the eggplant by rubbing it against a paper towel. Place the eggplants into a coated dish, and spread olive oil onto the eggplant as well. Layer the mozzarella cheese onto the eggplant, and then layer more eggplant on top of the cheese, this time covering it with ricotta and sauce. The last layer should be eggplant. Sprinkle the top of the casserole with cheese, and cook for a half hour.

Prep Instructions:

Place ¼ of the eggplant into 4 meal prep containers for a hearty and delicious meal. This lasagna will stay fresh in the refrigerator for up to 5 days.

Vegan Recipe 8: Tofu with a Kick

Prep time: 10 minutes; **Cook time:** 15 minutes; **Serving Size:** 8 ounces of tofu; **Serves:** 4; **Calories:** 400; **Total Fat:** 30 g; **Protein:** 25 g; **Total Carbs:** 10 g; **Net Carbs:** 5 g; **Sugar:** 3 g; **Fiber:** 5 g;

Ingredients:

- 16 ounces firm tofu
- 8 teaspoons sesame oil
- 8 tablespoons coconut oil
- 16 tablespoons chili sauce
- 8 tablespoons sesame seeds
- 2 teaspoons of each: garlic powder, chili powder, onion powder, paprika, salt and pepper
- 16 tablespoons soy sauce
- 1 cup almonds, sliced

Directions:

Dry the tofu with a paper towel, pressing on it to make sure that all of the moisture is removed. Slice the tofu into chunks, and then heat the coconut oil on a stovetop pan. Mix in the tofu and heat for roughly 2 minutes on each side. You want the tofu to be crispy. Mix in the sliced almonds and continue to heat. Add the spices and 4 tablespoons of sesame seeds. Mix the water and soy sauce together, before pouring into the pan. Make sure that all of the tofu is coated evenly.

Prep Instructions:

Divide equal amounts of this recipe into 4 meal prep containers and place inside refrigerator for up to 5 days.

Vegan Recipe 9: Mexi-Cauliflower Taco Bowl

Prep time: 15 minutes; **Cook time:** 15 minutes; **Serving Size:** 1.5 cups cauliflower mix; **Serves:** 8; **Calories:** 115; **Total Fat:** 6.4 g; **Protein:** 8 g; **Total Carbs:** 3 g; **Net Carbs:** 1.6 g; **Sugar:** 1 g; **Fiber:** 1.4 g;

Ingredients:

- 12 cups cauliflower pieces
- 4 tablespoons cilantro
- 2 tablespoons chili powder
- 4 teaspoons cumin
- 3 cups bell pepper
- 8 tomatoes, diced
- 4 jalapenos, diced
- 12 minced garlic cloves
- 4 onions, diced
- 4 tablespoons olive oil
- Pepper and salt, as needed

Directions:

In a food processor, cut up the cauliflower until it's in spall pieces. You want the cauliflower to look like rice. In a pan, combine the onions, garlic, and jalapenos. Wait until the onion is clear before adding the tomatoes, paprika, salt and cumin powder. Add the bell peppers and finally the cauliflower. Cook until the cauliflower is soft, about ten minutes.

Prep Instructions:

Deseeding the jalapenos will make this recipe less spicy. It's best to freeze this recipe if you're going to eat it right away, as cauliflower can develop a unique odor. Place in meal prep containers and refrigerate for no more than 3 days.

Vegan Recipe 10: Crazy-Good Cauliflower Grilled Cheese

Prep time: 10 minutes; **Cook time:** 15 minutes; **Serving Size:** 1 sandwich; **Serves:** 6; **Calories:** 380; **Total Fat:** 30 g; **Protein:** 25 g; **Total Carbs:** 10 g; **Net Carbs:** 3 g; **Sugar:** 3 g; **Fiber:** 7 g;

Ingredients:

- ¼ teaspoon pepper
- 1 tablespoon butter
- 1 cup cheddar cheese
- 9 cups cauliflower pieces
- 3 eggs, beaten
- 1.5 cups mozzarella cheese
- ½ teaspoon salt

Directions:

Heat oven to 450 degrees Fahrenheit. Place parchment paper on a cookie sheet and spray with nonstick cooking spray. Next, in a food processor, place the cauliflower. Once chopped, place into the microwave and cook for 8 minutes. This will help to dry it out. If it's not dry once microwaved, place it onto a towel and get rid of the rest of the moisture. Once dry, combine with egg, mozzarella, salt and pepper in a bowl. Make the "bread" squares by forming squares of cauliflower. Place in the oven and bake for 15 short minutes. On the stove, take the cauliflower bread and butter it before cooking. Drizzle this slice with cheese, before placing a cauliflower slice on top of it and also coating with butter. Cook for 1.5 minutes on each side.

Prep Instructions:

You can also opt to bake these sandwiches in the oven at 450 degrees Fahrenheit if you're not looking to fry the sandwich in butter. Doing this will make the sandwich less greasy and overall healthier. Divide grilled cheese sandwiches into 6 meal prep containers and place inside refrigerator for up to 5 days.

CONCLUSION

Congratulations on making it to the end of this book! Hopefully, this book has provided you with valuable information regarding why you should be considering implementing a ketogenic and meal prepping diet into your life. As you move towards becoming a healthier you, keep in mind the phrase, "Progress not Perfection". If you take small steps towards the greater goal that you have of cleaning up your diet, there's no doubt that these small steps will eventually turn into an entire lifestyle change. Be consistent, stay dedicated to your intentions, and try not to be too hard on yourself. At the end of the day, these are the types of things you should be trying to keep in mind.

The next step is to choose your favorite recipes that were documented in this book and try them out for a week yourself. Prep all of your food on either a Sunday or a Monday, and try not to deviate or eat out after you cook up these recipes. Generally speaking, it takes about 3 weeks for a consistent habit to form, so try to be particularly disciplined during these first three weeks. If you remain consistent, what you're going to find is that after the three-week period, things are going to become a bit easier for you.

Finally, if you enjoyed this book, then I'd like to ask you for a favor, would you be kind enough to leave a review for this book on Amazon? It'd be greatly appreciated!

Thank you and good luck on your health journey!

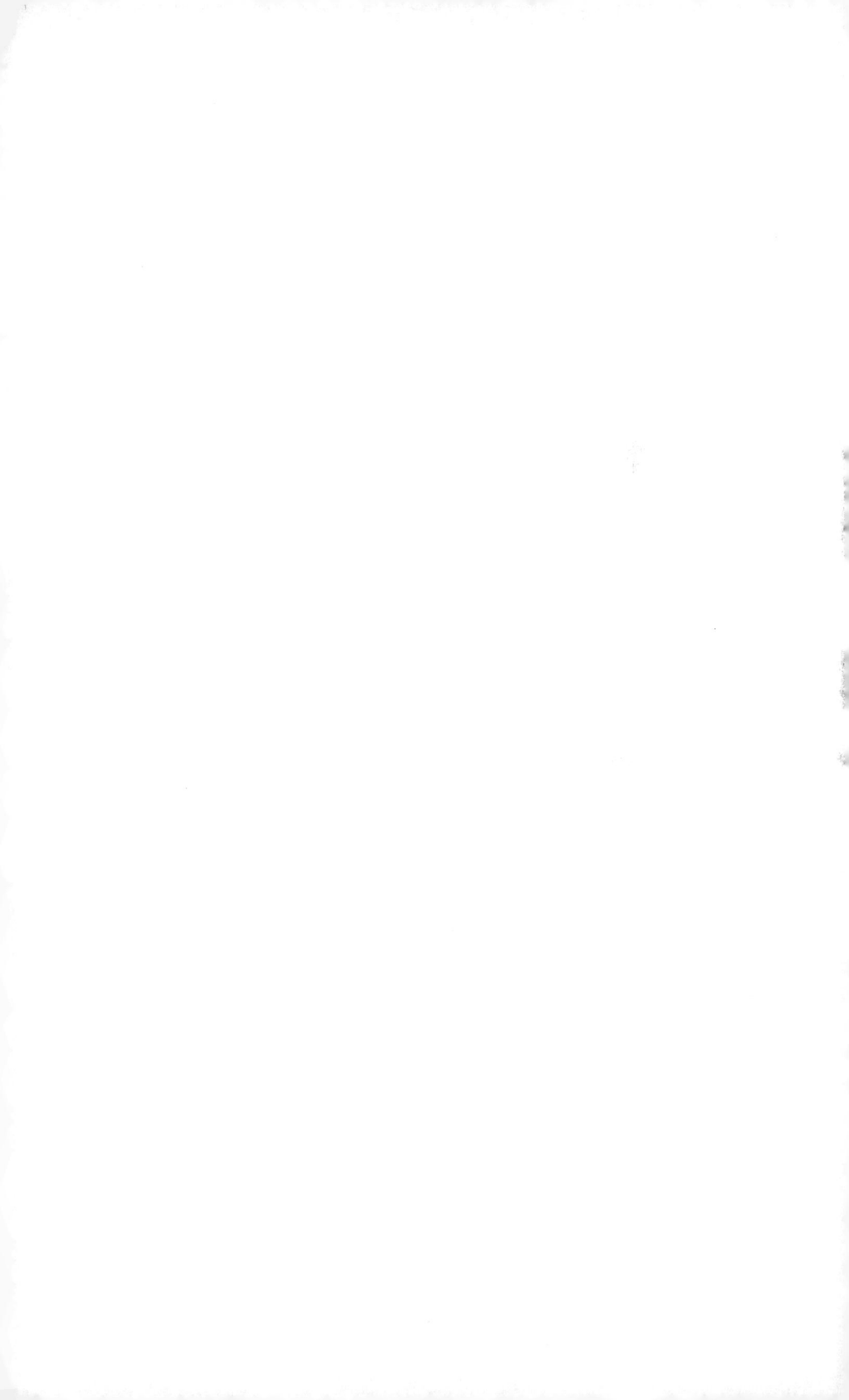

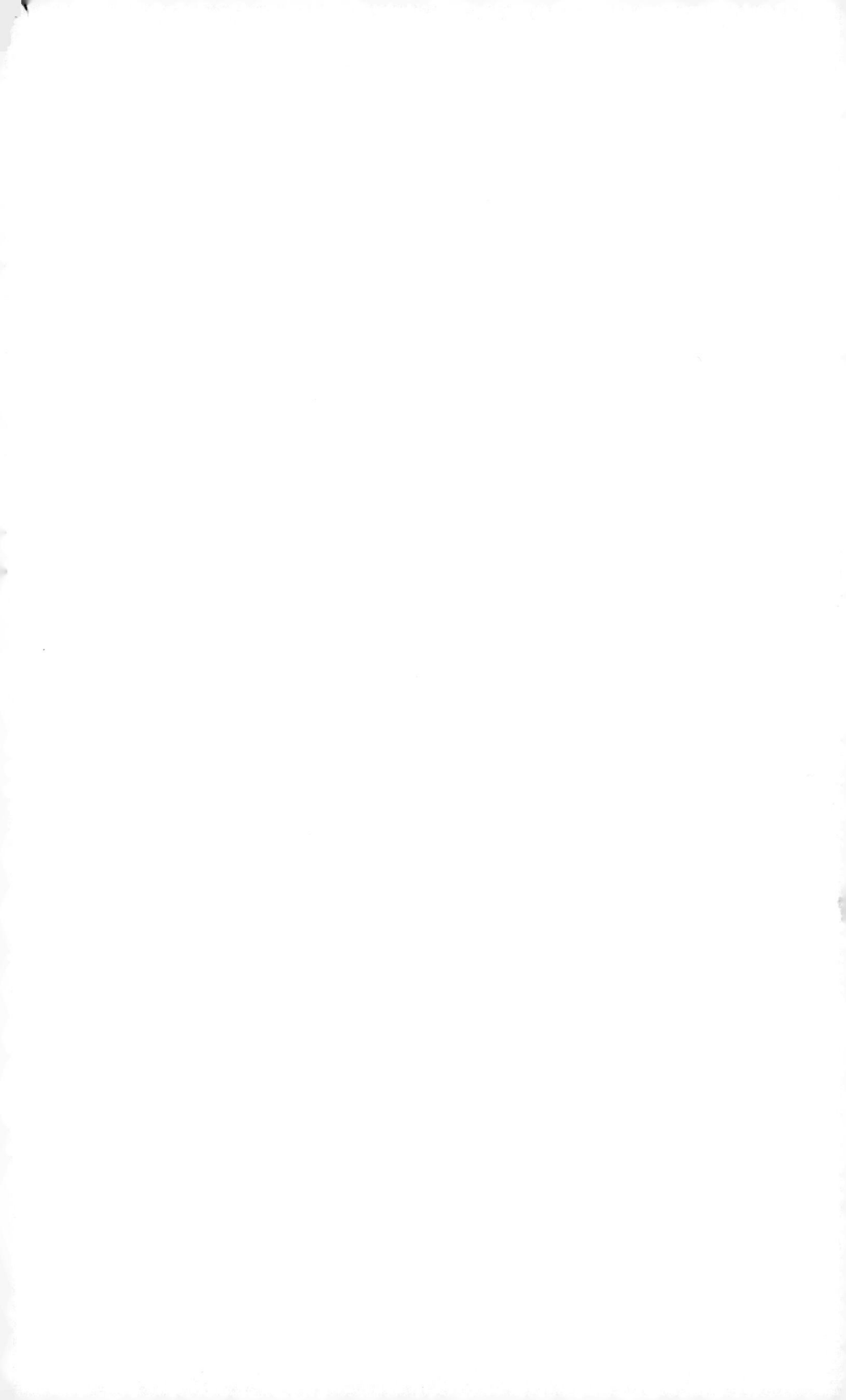

Printed in Great Britain
by Amazon